SURVIVAL OF ILLNESS

Dorothy W. Smith, R.N., Ed.D., F.A.A.N., earned her B.S.N. from Cornell University–New York Hospital School of Nursing, her M.A. from New York University, and her Ed.D. from Teachers College, Columbia University. She is a professor of nursing at The College of Nursing, Rutgers University, Newark, New Jersey, and has written books and articles dealing with nursing and nursing education, among which are *Care of the Adult Patient* (with Carol Germain), *Pharmacology and Drug Therapy in Nursing* (with Morton Rodman), and *Perspectives on Clinical Teaching.* An article based on this research study appeared in the *American Journal of Nursing* in March 1979 titled "Survivors of Serious Illness."

Contributors

Doreen Anne Kolditz, R.N., Ed.D., was awarded her doctoral degree from Columbia University's Teachers College in 1975. She is assistant director, Loeb Center for Nursing and Rehabilitation, Montefiore Hospital and Medical Center, New York.

Rose Ann Naughton, R.N., Ed.D., received her doctorate from Teachers College, Columbia University in 1975. She is associate professor of nursing at Molloy College, Rockville Center, New York.

SURVIVAL OF ILLNESS
Implications for Nursing

151 634815

Dorothy W. Smith, R.N., Ed.D., F.A.A.N.

Contributors

Doreen Anne Kolditz, R.N., Ed.D.
Rose Ann Naughton, R.N., Ed.D.

SPRINGER PUBLISHING COMPANY
New York

Springer Publishing Company, Inc.
200 Park Avenue South
New York, New York 10003

81 82 83 84 85 / 10 9 8 7 6 5 4 3 2 1

Library of Congress Cataloging in Publication Data

Smith, Dorothy W
  Survival of illness.

  Bibliography: p.
  Includes index.
    1. Nursing—Psychological aspects. 2. Sick—
Psychology. 3. Convalescence. 4. Rehabilitation
nursing. I. Kolditz, Doreen Anne, joint author.
II. Naughton, Rose Ann, joint author. III. Title.
RT86.S62   616'.001'9   80-27149
ISBN 0-8261-2870-X
ISBN 0-8261-2871-8 (pbk.)

To my daughters,
Shannon and Helena

Contents

Preface

Many people are questioning our culture's focus on the unlimited potential of science to maintain health and cure illness. Increasing emphasis is being placed on the patient's role in maintaining health and in participating in and fostering recovery when illness occurs. Meditation and biofeedback are two examples of ways in which clients are encouraged to help themselves. At the same time, many practitioners of nursing and medicine have maintained an emphasis on the patient as a passive recipient of care, and have confined their practice predominantly to technical aspects designed to alter pathophysiologic responses. Important as this aspect of care is, it is but one facet of the healing process. This book emphasizes understanding of the psychological aspects of the survival and recovery processes, and addresses the role nurses can play both in assisting patients to help themselves to recover and in fostering psychological growth as a consequence of illness.

The book is based on two studies: one focuses on medical–surgical and psychiatric and alcoholic patients who have survived an acute serious illness, the other on patients recovering from abdominal surgery. Both studies emphasize patients' subjective experiences with survival and recovery, and raise questions regarding the role of the nurse, stressing the importance of professional nursing care during recovery from illness. All data has been carefully disguised to protect patients' identities, and the health care institutions are not identified. Although the implications of the studies relate to nursing, the studies themselves may also be of interest to other health care professionals.

Many colleagues helped with this project, and it would be impossible to list all their names here. Special thanks are expressed to Dr. Barbara Callaway, Dr. Beverly Bowns, and Dr. Shirley Smoyak of Rutgers University; Dr. Carol Germain of the University of Pennsylvania, and Ms. Grace Phelan and Ms. Gloria Odin. Special thanks are also due the Busch Foundation for financial support of this project.

I sincerely appreciate the participation of Dr. Ursula Springer and Ms. Helen Behnke of Springer Publishing Company. They gave much encouragement, help, and a great deal of patience.

Dorothy W. Smith

Chapter 1

Introduction

The two studies on which this book is based represent efforts to explore the relevance to nursing of the literature on the process of survival and recovery. The emphasis is on the need for nurses to understand that process. Survival may be viewed as an end stage in recovery from acute illness or from an acute episode during chronic illness. Concepts of survival are most relevant to those illnesses that the patient perceives as serious or life-threatening.

Survival is most often thought of in relation to such mass disasters as floods, fires, earthquakes, and, at its extreme, survival of concentration camps. Concepts of survival, widely discussed in the literature, also have relevance for individuals who undergo acute illness, an acute episode of chronic illness, or an experience with major surgery. These people, too, may be viewed as survivors. Utilization of concepts from the literature on survival in the care of these patients may help some of them grow through the experience of illness and may assist nurses to broaden their understanding and their practice. Although nurses currently use concepts from crisis theory and crisis intervention in their practice, the literature on survival has been less extensively applied.

Perhaps this difference in utilization of the literature reflects the somewhat negative connotation of the word *survival*. Des Pres (1976) has pointed out that survival is often described as "mere survival," when, in fact, it is the basis of continued life from which all other opportunities for further human development flow. Survival often has a positive connotation when it is linked with heroism. However, this linkage removes it from the experience of ordinary people who, as described by Camus (1948), are not necessarily heroic, but are doing what has to be done to maintain life with as much dignity and decency as possible. Perhaps many patients resemble Camus's description: overtaken by illness, they are doing what they can in a daily way in order to survive. Illness is often not dramatic nor its endurance necessarily heroic. It is simply part of life. Like the inevitability of death, the possibility of illness is frequently denied in modern society. Such denial may be especially easy in situations in which the incidence of illness has indeed been vastly reduced. Despite having less illness to deal with in our society, those who are ill may find less tolerance for their condition, and less emphasis upon possibly learning from it, in a culture that holds health as a central value.

Like other health professions, nursing emphasizes both prevention of illness and care during illness to assist the individual to regain health. It is natural to view illness as something to prevent and from which to recover. With this orientation, however, it is easy to deemphasize the personal growth an individual can gain through experiencing illness. Conversely, recognizing illness as part of life (however much one wishes to avoid it) helps an individual to consider what may be gained from going through the experience. The longer one lives, the greater the possibility of illness. The nurse who views life as best when untouched by illness may especially value youth, where the possibility of this state is greatest. On the other hand, the nurse who also appreciates the varied ways in which people can develop through illness and misfortune (as well as through protection from these events) may view the process of aging with greater tolerance.

Survival is linked to recovery. Recovery is a dynamic process that looks to the future. In contrast, some descriptions of recovery emphasize that it is a return (to the extent possible) to a former state. Because experiences can change individuals, the patient may be expected to have changed in some ways as a result of going through illness. The concept of recovery as a return to a former state does not give adequate recognition to this possibility, and unnecessarily limits nursing's role in assisting patients to experience personal growth as an aspect of the illness experience. Thus, a predominant focus upon whether the patient can walk as well as he or she used to may crowd out the equally important question of how the patient wants to use his or her abilities and energy in the future. What goals seem most important to the patient? Are his or her goals unchanged? Whatever the answers, it can be helpful for the patient to begin to explore such questions. It may be an especially important assessment for those patients who are facing either some limitation imposed by the illness or a heightened awareness of limitations, such as of mortal life, or of physical and emotional energy. Predominant references to and comparisons with past abilities are useful in establishing baseline data. However, if discussions with the patient about possible changes in values and goals are not included, the possibility of the natural and spontaneous personal growth that can occur as a result of surviving illness is diminished. A focus on the past may also lessen the nurse's awareness that such negative emotions as apathy, constriction of interests, and persistent anger and bitterness may be present.

Acute illness, recovery, and survival are on a continuum, and are related to one another. In the acute stage,

intensive effort at life support, which considers both physio-
logic and emotional needs, prepares the way for the patient
to move toward recovery. Helping the recovering patient
both to regain capacities temporarily lost and to assess possible limitations and possible personal growth prepares the
way for a positive survival experience. The illness–survival
cycle can be repeated many times in the course of life. The
way the experience is handled by the patient and by those
who care for him or her affects subsequent experiences.

Society and the health care system differ greatly in the
amount of support they give at these various stages. The
needs of the patient during the acute phase are often dramatic. Society is most generous with support and care at this
time. In its relationship with the patient society emphasizes
nurturance, relative passivity and dependence of the patient, with decision making largely in the hands of professionals. Recovery and survival also present demands, but
they are not usually as compellingly visible. Care during the
recovery phase may be deemphasized with such comments
as, "He can take care of himself now." Survival concerns,
such as consideration of how the illness has affected the
patient's view of himself or herself and others and his or
her values and priorities, may be disregarded. Not all
change is positive. One can survive with bitterness, apathy,
and constriction of interests. This is not only a personal loss,
but a social loss as well. The loss of workers who no longer
have the energy and interest to give to their jobs, parents
who can no longer cope with their children, and spouses
who cannot maintain the give-and-take of a close human
relationship, represent not only personal losses, but also
losses to society. Perhaps some of these negative outcomes
may be lessened by conscious, thoughtful attention to the
existential aspects of the illness experience.

Nursing has focused on acute illness both in practice
and in nursing education. In addition, nursing has empha-

sized the use of time tables that specify when various outcomes are expected as a result of nursing intervention.
While appropriate for such aspects of nursing as learning
transfer from bed to wheelchair, there are processes for
which such specific time tables are inappropriate. These
processes unfold within the patient and can be facilitated by
nurses and other professionals, but are somewhat unpre-
dictable. One cannot predict that by a certain date a patient
will accept a major change in body image, and consider that
problem solved. Rather, the nurse should work with the
patient to help him or her achieve this goal, while recognizing it as an ongoing process that may seem solved at one
time, only to emerge again later, perhaps in response to
some future life event.

How feasible is it for nurses to involve themselves with
these aspects of care? Discussions such as this can become
part of group teaching programs. Nurses, especially those
in private practice, can incorporate this aspect of care into
work with individual patients and with families. The more
independently and broadly the nurse views his or her role,
the more possible it becomes to encompass aspects of nursing designed to assist the patient toward a positive survival
experience.

Another factor limiting the role of the nurse in relation
to survival is his or her position in the health care hierarchy.
Until very recently, nurses have been restricted largely to
following physicians' orders and to maintaining the smooth
functioning of a health care institution. Neither of these
endeavors is likely to place much emphasis on survival
issues or, in fact, on any aspect of creativity and autonomy
by the nurse. An important change is gradually occurring in
nursing, however, in that the nurse is gaining greater autonomy and capacity for decision making. With this change
comes an increasing opportunity to address the patient care
issues that are relevant to nursing and that are often seri-

ously neglected. The recovery and survival concerns addressed in this book are two examples.

Nurses who creatively extend their practice enhance opportunities for their own personal growth. Because such human experiences as illness and recovery are universal, the nurses who are open to patients' experiences and who are actively involved in helping patients cope with these experiences find that their own lives have been enriched.

Chapter 2

Some Concepts from the Literature

Many authors have discussed survival experiences and their impact on future life. Literature on survival has been especially plentiful since World War II and deals with survival of such natural disasters as earthquakes, fires, and floods, and such man-made disasters as war, German and Russian concentration camps, and forced migrations. Themes highlighted in the literature include changes in basic values, reordering of priorities, guilt, and psychic numbing. Studies of survival of illness have also been done and will be discussed later in this chapter.

What relevance has this literature for nursing? Although differences between the survival experience of patients and of those experiencing mass disaster are apparent, there are commonalities in the process of survival. After an earthquake or flood large groups of people are involved in a shared catastrophe. Usually society responds by discussing the event, classifying the victims as survivors, and bringing aid, and the event is perceived as extraordinary. In contrast, survival of illness is a relatively common experience, despite the fact that each individual undergoing it usually perceives it as an extraordinary one. Although others are having similar experiences simultaneously, the patient is treated primarily as one individual, rather than as part of a group. Thus the patient is admitted for treatment, cared for, and discharged according to an individualized time schedule and plan of therapy that reflects his or her particular need and experience.

Despite these obvious differences, it is helpful to consider the relevance of concepts of survival to the experiences of patients recovering from serious illness. Understanding the survival experience more fully can help nurses assist patients to use the experience for personal growth; nurses may also be able to help patients avoid the persistent psychic numbing and constriction of personal growth that can also occur in the process of survival.

Robert Jay Lifton has written extensively about Vietnam warriors as survivors and about survival after the bombing of Hiroshima (1973, 1974, 1976). Some of the themes and concepts presented by Lifton are:

- Touching death as a condition for new growth or for psychic numbing and constriction of life.
- Considering survival in relation to systems theory. Survivors have lost power in the system and are hurt by it. Those who have gained power have a stake in keeping survivors powerless to avoid evoking their own guilt and to prevent retaliation by them. Keeping survivors in a dependent and marginal position serves to justify hurting them; they are viewed as outside the group and different from the dominant group.
- Feeling guilty, considering that one's survival may have been at the expense of others who did not survive; wondering if the experience was one's own fault, or was merited by past mistakes and failings.
- Seeking new ways of living and experiencing; making the rest of one's life count more; seeking renewal and new values and opportunities: rebirth.

While Lifton discusses both positive and negative aspects of the survivor experience, Kai Erikson (1976), in his description of the Buffalo Creek flood, emphasizes the prevalence of psychic numbing and a loss of a sense of community among survivors. He notes the failure of local and national agencies to support community relationships.

Many writers have described the impact of concentration camp experiences on victims and victims' children. Neiderland (1961), uses the term *survivor syndrome* to describe the following group of symptoms:

- chronic anxiety and depression
- nightmares
- guilt due to surviving while others died
- psychosomatic disorders
- loneliness, isolation, lack of pleasure

Phillips (1978) describes the problems of children of camp survivors this way:

- overprotection of children by parents
- inculcation of guilt into children for having a better life than their parents had
- extreme suspicion of the Gentile world; limiting children to the home and to very narrow contacts outside the home
- expectation that the children will vindicate parents' suffering

Muhlen (1962) has described the process by which Jews reentered life in Germany after World War II and the many problems that arose, such as idealization of the Jews and the inability of Jews to respond to gestures of acceptance following their victimization. His emphasis is on the gradual resuming of relationships and the slow healing following such a massive trauma. Rubenstein (1966) has discussed many aspects of survival of the concentration camps, emphasizing the importance of guilt (assumption of guilt by Jews for the death of Jesus and, therefore, the necessity for punishment by the Holocaust) and the scapegoating of Jews in their relationships with Germans.

Other writers have indicated some positive aspects of survival of the Holocaust. Terrence Des Pres (1976) stresses the sense of community and the interdependence that flourished among victims despite conditions of extreme suffering. Des Pres states that:

- Survival under such extreme circumstances had to be a group effort with emphasis on mutual support, gift giving, and concern for others as well as for oneself.
- Loss of dignity and loss of privacy are among the most powerful forces lessening the will to live.
- The process of healing is a slow turning back to life, often initiated by some caring contact with another person.
- Survivors' priorities are, and have to be, different from those of people in other circumstances.

Whereas survival is often described as "mere survival," Des Pres points out that survival is a worthy goal in itself. Surviving to bear witness, to testify so that others may know what happened and try to prevent recurrence, is an important goal among many survivors. De Pres also indicates that the concept of death as heroic is sometimes false. Death can prevent confronting a situation, whereas survival means that the person is present and thus has the opportunity to cope. Des Pres emphasizes the importance of stubbornly preventing one's own dissolution, and of holding some parts of the self inviolate despite degrading experiences.

Dimsdale (1978) discusses survival within the context of concentration camp experience. He describes the following coping methods used by survivors:

- focusing on the good or the positive in the situation
- emphasis on the purpose of survival
- psychological protection: insulating oneself from overwhelming stress
- mastery through expression of autonomy in some aspects of life
- will to live
- summoning hope
- group support

Bruno Bettelheim (1960) has described the initial shock of camp life, noting that the greatest number of deaths occur during that period. He describes his own process of learning to survive in an overwhelmingly threatening and hostile situation, stressing his struggle to maintain individuality and to avoid being absorbed into a destructive system.

Des Pres and Lifton stress that civilization and technology obscure the bare facts of life and reduce our consciousness of ourselves as biological creatures. These facts include vulnerability to injury and illness, and the inevitability of death. Des Pres describes the sensitivity to beauty that is often intensified among those whose survival is threatened. He poignantly describes the heightened awareness of the beauty of the stars among those who were staggering under a burden of starvation, illness, and exhaustion from heavy labor. Des Pres further states that in meeting extraordinary demands daily, some survivors became more fundamentally human, more clear-sighted about priorities and values, more firmly rooted in the biological and social facts of existence, and less vulnerable to the various deceptions offered by society and modern technology.

Kübler-Ross (1969) has called attention to the harmful effects of the deception involved in the denial of death. Her writings indicate that awareness of death is important in improving the quality of life.

Mitscherlich and Mitscherlich (1975) emphasize the rigidity of role taking that occurs in modern society. Individual growth may be hampered by acquiescence to the demands of various groups that particular roles be played. Extreme crisis can strip away conventional roles. To the extent that an individual has not developed an inner sense of self, the loss of conventional roles can leave a feeling of loss of identity, or nothingness. On the other hand, the crisis can spur the individual to find a more enduring sense of identity.

Survival of life-threatening illness constitutes severe stress. Horowitz (1976), in discussing stress responses, indicates that the following stages occur:

- phase of initial recognition—outcry
- phase of denial and numbing
- mixed phase of denial and intrusive repetition
- further ideational and emotional processes to integrate the experience

He stresses the importance of support in assisting the individual to move through the various stages, so that he or she does not become immobilized in an early stage of the process. These stages are similar to those described by Kübler-Ross (1969), among patients who are confronting death:

- denial and isolation
- anger
- bargaining
- depression
- acceptance

Both authors stress the importance of supporting the patient as he or she moves through these stages, of identifying and respecting the stages, and of recognizing a patient's slowness or inability (at that time) to progress from one stage to another.

Survival of immigrants who were forced by extreme poverty to come to the United States has been described by Oscar Handlin (1973). He describes many of the immigrants' ways of coping, such as utilization of support networks and flexibility in the fact of radical changes in their experience. Handlin also describes the wearing down, fatigue, and loss of resilience that prevented some immigrants from continuing their migration toward more desirable locations and circumstances, and instead, left them trapped in the slums of large cities. The situation of patients who have survived a serious illness, but who lack the energy and optimism needed to achieve a higher level of recovery, is analogous.

Aaron Antonovsky (1979) provides a related but somewhat different view concerning survival. He questions why, in an environment full of stressors and threats to health, more people are not sick. He postulates that resistance is a crucial factor. After considering such classic aspects of resistance as nutrition, rest, and exercise, he indicates that resistance involves other factors as well. He believes that an important aspect of resistance is a sense of coherence—a sense of confidence that one's environment is predictable and that things will work out as well as can be expected. According to this view, an individual with a stable family and community and with a stable sense of values and optimistic beliefs has a greater chance of survival than one who lacks these attributes.

Studies have been performed on the development and survival of illness. Simonton and Simonton have studied personality factors in relation to development of and recovery from cancer (Simonton, 1974). They state that personality is one risk factor in the development of cancer. Cancer-prone individuals experience pain in close interpersonal relationships, are especially shaken by the loss of a loved person, and are vulnerable to depression. The authors also state that cancer patients whose faith and will to live are kindled have an increased chance of recovery.

Booth (1973) has also done studies of cancer patients. He emphasizes the importance of faith and hope in recovering from cancer and describes seemingly miraculous cures that have occurred. Booth points out that these spontaneous cures are largely ignored by the medical profession, as are the psychological aspects of cancer. LeShan (1959) has carried out similar studies of cancer patients, treating personality as a factor in susceptibility to and recovery from cancer.

Bilodeau and Hackett have studied patients who survived myocardial infarction (1971). They raise many points concerning the recovery of these patients, including:

- •the importance of denial in helping the patient to survive the acute episode, as well as the importance of helping the patient to deal with his or her denial when the acute episode is over
- •the necessity for mourning as an aspect of recovery from any serious illness
- •the constructive management of depression following the acute episode
- •the necessity of including families in the rehabilitation process
- •the value of education for patients and families
- •the usefulness of groups as a modality for support and education
- •the importance of morale and self-confidence to recovery

In relation to survival of illness, these studies stress some of the same concepts that Des Pres has discussed concerning survivors of concentration camps. Des Pres emphasizes the relationship between emotional and physical states and the importance of both for survival. He points out the importance of continuing to be part of a human network and of not giving in—points that are also discussed in relation to survival of cancer and myocardial infarction.

What relevance may these concepts have for nursing? The literature on survival provides a useful conceptual framework for understanding patients' communications about their illness and recovery experiences. The importance of listening to and talking with patients has been stressed in nursing. Understanding some of the themes that frequently arise among those with similar experiences can alert the nurse to such themes in the communications of patients. The following are examples of themes that may be relevant to patients who have survived a serious illness.

• *Touching death, hitting bottom:* Do patients who have had a brush with death sometimes see values and priorities more clearly, as though they suddenly have a different perception of these priorities? A brush with death can sometimes bring home vulnerability, in a creature-like way, to hurt and to illness. While this can be anxiety-provoking, it may also be reassuring in the sense that a reality, which has always been there but which has been previously denied, is acknowledged. Patients may say, "It can happen to me; it has happened to me; now I have a different view of myself and of my life." Does the patient express apathy and hopelessness, or persistent bitterness?

• *Systems:* During illness, patients must relinquish some of their usual roles. In addition, some illnesses such as psychiatric illness, are very stigmatizing. How does the identified patient become part of work relationships and family relationships again? Once viewed as outside the inner circle of work life and home life, reentry may be difficult. The individual who has been through a survival experience may, in fact, be viewed as deviant from his or her work group and family group because of changes in his values and priorities and because he may be less open to such manipulations as flattery. The fact of acknowledging death can place usual office politics and pressures in a different perspective and, while liberating for the individual, may serve to isolate him or her from groups that do not share his or her values. On the other hand, do patient and family now share more concerning their values as a result of the illness experience, and are they developing closer relationships?

• *Guilt:* How often do patients feel that their illness is their fault, and that through this fault they are hurting not only themselves but their families and colleagues? How much has the recent emphasis on health maintenance and individual responsibility added to guilt when an individual becomes ill? How many times do we hear patients say, "I did this to myself" or "This happened as a punishment"?

• *Loss of privacy and dignity:* Much has been written about these aspects of patienthood. How do these losses affect patients as they enter the process of recovery? What measures help patients get over their feelings about intrusion and lessened control?

• *Group support:* How can recovering patients be helped by other patients, and how can they give help? How can opportunities for such group experience be maximized? What environmental factors facilitate group support?

• *Focus on the positive:* Although much has been written about the importance of helping patients deal with denial, many nurses have intuitively recognized that patients need some protection from the massively anxiety-provoking experiences they undergo during the acute phase of illness. Research, such as that done by Bilodeau and Hackett (1971), supports the commonsense view that confrontation is not always desirable or useful, and that it may even be hazardous, as among patients suffering an acute myocardial infarction. Timing is important; patients need time to recover somewhat from the severe physiological and psychological effects of serious illness before they can be expected to confront the reality of what has happened to them.

• *Stages of experience:* A great deal has been written about stages of experience in relation to grief and loss. Illness and recovery, too, have their stages. How often do we attempt to telescope these stages into much less time, in response to the emphasis on a shortened hospital stay? It is likely that many patients leave the hospital in a stage of denial. What plans are made for follow-up care to help them move through this stage?

• *Mastery, autonomy:* Survivors often indicate the importance of having some sphere of their lives uninvaded by the threatening experience. What opportunities are there for patients to keep some aspects of their lives free from the illness experience, as by continuing a hobby or an aspect of their work?

• *Healing:* While a skin incision heals relatively quickly, feelings take time to heal. Do we expect patients, once discharged from the hospital, to be more ready to resume stressful activities than may be possible? How much emphasis do we give to factors that enhance the psychological healing process, such as unhurried contact with nature and opportunities for contact with beauty?

• *Will to live:* Survival comes at the price of energy and effort. There is the possibility of loss of resilience and will, of succumbing to the process of being worn down, and of relinquishing hope. Having a reason for survival is important in summoning hope and strength. Health care services typically diminish after the acute phase is over. The patient, however, may not have the energy and other personal resources to continue recovery without outside assistance.

Although experiencing illness can foster personal growth, it can also lead to bitterness, apathy, and constriction

of interests. How many patients never recover psychologi-
cally, even though they survive physically, from the effects of
myocardial infarction or a stroke? How often do families say,
"He's just never been the same since his heart attack, but the
doctor says he has recovered." Such a comment raises the
issue of professional responsibility not only for physical survival but also for assisting the patient with psychological healing. Too often this aspect of care is viewed as a frill, as something to be considered after the important aspects of care
have been completed, rather than as a central concern. Ideally, this is a task for all health professionals, especially those
who work with patients in later stages after the acute crisis
has passed. How can nurses participate in this helping process? Is such help just one more thing to do on the part of
those who are already overburdened, or is it a basic framework within which the nursing role can be conceptualized?

The process of recovery is related to survival. How do
patients view their own recovery? What do they perceive as
helpful in recovery? How do they view their own role in the
process? What kinds of actions by staff are viewed as facilitating recovery? In an effort to understand these questions,
a study was undertaken of patients recovering from serious
illness—illness that realistically could lead to feelings of
vulnerability to death or hitting bottom. The next chapter
deals with a description of the study.

Chapter 3

Study of Survivors of Serious Illness: Description and Findings

Subjects

Eighty-six patients who were recovering from medical–surgical, psychiatric, and alcoholic conditions were interviewed. Patients were selected whose illness was acute and severe, and who had strong likelihood of recovery. There were 44 medical–surgical, 31 psychiatric, and 11 alcoholic patients in the study.*

Patient interviews were conducted in two settings: a voluntary community hospital and an inpatient service of a community mental health center. All patients were adults, aged 18 to 83. Diagnoses of the medical–surgical patients were as follows.

Diagnosis	Number of patients
myocardial infarction	12
fracture of leg and hip	10
herniorrhaphy	5

*Categories reflected those of the hospitals. In other hospitals, alcoholic patients might have been classified with medical–surgical or psychiatric patients, rather than separately.

radical mastectomy	4
hysterectomy	3
cholecystectomy	2
asthma	1
laminectomy	1
Stokes–Adams syndrome, pacemaker insertion	1
appendectomy for ruptured appendix	1
cerebrovascular accident	1
bowel resection	1
pneumonia	1
bleeding peptic ulcer	1

Diagnoses of psychiatric patients were as follows.

Diagnosis	Number of patients
acute schizophrenia	15
acute depression	8
acute anxiety state	5
obsessive–compulsive reaction	3

The 76 white patients and 10 black patients in the study were predominantly middle class. They were interviewed within 2 or 3 days of their discharge from the hospital. Three patients were interviewed again after their return home. While a follow-up interview of this type would have been desirable with all patients, it was not feasible due to time limitations.

The Interview

Tape-recorded interviews that lasted approximately 45 minutes were conducted. Patients were assured that their responses would be among those given by at least 50 other people and that their names or other identifying data would not be used. In addition to questions likely to elicit survivor themes, patients were asked about the experience of recovery in an effort to evaluate their feelings about the survival experience within the context of such daily aspects of recovery as self-care and care by staff. The following questions about the experience of recovery were asked:

1. Tell me about your illness and your recovery.
2. Are there ways in which your values, goals, and priorities have changed since the period before your illness?
3. What do you do to help yourself recover?
4. Are there things that you do, that you notice hinder your recovery?
5. What approaches by nurses and other staff help you recover?
6. Do nurses and other staff do things that hinder your recovery?
7. Do you feel any differently toward other people now than you did before your illness? If so, in what ways?
8. What else would you like to tell me about your recovery?

Varied Diagnoses

Patients' conditions differ, of course, in significant ways. The experience of myocardial infarction is different from that of radical mastectomy, and these conditions in turn differ from depression and schizophrenia. Alcoholic patients are viewed as having similar dynamics that are different from those of nonalcoholic patients. However, in all patients there was the likelihood of experiencing a threat to their physical and or psychological survival. The feeling of hitting bottom, either in a physical or psychological sense, was a possibility for all of them. The study focused on the patient's experience of threat to his or her physical and/or psychological survival, on the effects of this threat on values, priorities, and relationships with others, and on his or her perceptions of recovery, rather than on particular diagnoses. Staff's perceptions of threat were not considered. On a busy medical–surgical unit many of these patients' conditions may be viewed by staff as routine, especially likely in the case of surgical patients.

Limitations of the Study

Patients were interviewed only once. Thus other aspects of their survivor experience, which may have come up during a continuing relationship and further interviews, were not elicited. Because patients' responses to these questions may change significantly after being involved in family and work life, it would be desirable to do a follow-up study at a later time, such as a year after the initial interview. This would be useful in determining the extent to which these patients changed their responses after they became immersed in the pressures of job and family life.

The study focused on individual patients. It would be useful to interview patients with their families, since families, too, are likely to experience changes in their values as a result of the illness of a close relative, and because changes in the patient's values and priorities will have an affect on his or her family.

Thus this study was exploratory, and was undertaken in the hope that further study will be possible by the author and by others.

While acknowledging the usefulness and desirability of

a follow-up study, changes that patients describe at the end of the period of hospitalization and before resumption of home and work responsibilities have relevance for nursing and will be discussed in Chapter 5.

Findings of the Study

Findings of the study will be discussed first in relation to survivor themes and then in relation to specific questions about recovery. Numbers of patients giving various responses are provided.

Responses of medical–surgical patients were quite different from those of alcoholic and psychiatric patients. Responses of the latter two groups of patients were very similar. This similarity of responses does not imply similarity of patients' conditions, however. Differences in responses among the three groups of patients will be discussed further in relation to their implications for nursing (see Chapter 5).

Survivor Themes

Most survivor themes were brought up in responses to the following questions:

• Are there ways in which your values, goals, and priorities have changed since the period before your illness?
• Do you feel differently toward other people now than you did before your illness?
• What else would you like to tell me about your recovery?

Values, goals, and priorities

Most (66%) medical–surgical patients spoke quickly and with feeling about changes in values and priorities, often prefacing their remarks with such comments as, "Isn't it strange that you should ask me that? I've been thinking about it a lot." Changes in values and priorities were quite similar among these patients. Typical responses were:

> I've put so much into my work, constantly hurrying and pushing. I've hardly had any time for myself. From now on I'm going to put more emphasis on enjoying life with my family.

> I'm thinking about whether the kind of work I do is what I really want, and also how I can make my home life better.

> I feel I've been brought up short and that I have to rethink a lot. Material things are now much less important to me. My health is now much more important, and my family is more important to me.

> I've been so caught up in the rat race, and in what everyone else thinks I should do and be. Now I'm thinking about what's right for me.

The similarity of responses was striking. Every medical–surgical patient who mentioned changes in values and priorities linked these changes to a heightened awareness of death and a sharp realization of his or her own limited lifespan. Typical comments were:

> It never occurred to me before that I could die. Now I know it will happen sometime even if it didn't happen this time.

> I realize I'm not going to live forever, and that has changed my views about a lot of things and my plans for the future.

Some medical–surgical patients (34%) stated that their values and goals had not changed. A typical comment was: "Nothing has changed in my life. My feelings and plans are the same as before." Patients who responded in this way either did not mention death or personal mortality at all, or they made such comments as, "It never once occurred to me I wouldn't get better. I just knew I would."

When responding to the question about values, goals, and priorities, most psychiatric and alcoholic patients (80%) stressed undervaluing themselves and their close personal relationships, especially those with their children, prior to therapy. They spoke frequently of trying to please everyone and of the lack of priorities in their lives. A typical comment was:

> I never put any value on myself and I guess I didn't value my kids either. I've got a lot of thinking to do about what's important to me, but I know one thing: I'm going to take better care of my kids.

Most of the psychiatric and alcoholic patients (80%) who expressed changes in values and priorities also mentioned fearing dissolution of their personalities and their abilities to cope with life. Typical comments were:

> My whole life had crumbled and I had crumbled too.

> I was at a complete dead end when I came here. I couldn't manage any more.

> I tried to kill myself because I couldn't see any use to living.

Some psychiatric and alcoholic patients (20%) expressed no changes in their values, goals, and priorities. None of these patients mentioned a sense of hitting bottom and most of them attributed hospitalization to the unwelcome and misguided intrusion of such others as families, employers, and physicians.

Thus, among all patients interviewed, awareness of death and/or a sense of hitting bottom were crucial to perceiving a need to change values, priorities, and goals. Changes were in the direction of humanistic rather than materialistic values, and toward more thoughtful, personal decisions about goals rather than toward uncritical acceptance of goals approved of by others. Some patients who had had severe myocardial infarctions described profound changes in their values and goals and a quickened sense of their mortality. Others who also had had severe infarctions described no such changes. Likewise, many surgical patients spoke of an awareness of death, its reality to them, and many changes in values and priorities, while others with similar conditions did not.

It is, of course, likely that the rate at which patients moved through the stages from denial to acceptance was one factor affecting responses. Some patients who denied these changes while still in the hospital may have experienced them after returning home. Rapidity of onset of illness may also have affected responses. Another factor affecting responses might be the differences in psychological development among the patients. It is reasonable to assume that some patients were more ready and able to move through denial to acceptance of the reality of illness than others. Also, as pointed out by Bilodeau and Hackett (1971), denial can help patients survive crisis. Thus some patients who never doubted that they would recover may have been helped through the crisis by this attitude. It is noteworthy, however, that personal growth experiences related to changes in values and priorities and to positive feelings toward others were closely associated with recognition of death as a personal reality and with concerns about hitting bottom.

Attitudes toward others

Most medical–surgical patients (70%) responded positively to the question "Do you feel any differently toward other people now than before your illness?" Those who gave this response had also described changes in values and goals and an awareness of death. They stated that they felt greater concern for others and a general sense of community with other people, with their families, and particularly with other patients. Typical comments were:

> I never knew what could happen to people. I find I care more about others, and I want to help them. I see so many who are worse off and I try to help.

> I feel less hemmed in by differences in age, sex, skin color. We're all in the same boat, trying to get well. I find myself talking to people I'd never talk to on the outside.

> One night I was hungry and kind of lonely and I went to the kitchenette for a snack. I met a man there, and we were both in our bathrobes, and we ate and told each other about our experiences and it didn't seem strange at all. It seemed the natural thing to do. There I was, telling him about my radical mastectomy.

A frequent comment among medical–surgical patients was how much better off they were than others. Interestingly, this remark was made most often by those who had been the sickest and who, therefore, seemed to have the least reason for making it.

Most psychiatric and alcoholic patients (86%) spoke of feeling more at ease with and more able to relate to others. Patients discussed this in terms of their therapy, particularly in relation to the groups they attended. However, probably because of the heavy emphasis on human relationships in their treatment and the expectation of this result, these patients' comments did not have the ring of surprise that was typical of the medical–surgical patients. In fact, most medical–surgical patients who reported changes in goals and values, as well as in attitudes toward others, spoke very spontaneously and with an air of surprise. Psychiatric and alcoholic patients, on the other hand, spoke in more matter-of-fact tones and attributed changes in themselves to the goals of their treatment programs.

When speaking of changes in attitudes toward others, 38% of the patients in all three groups described an unaccustomed feeling of being cared about and cared for by others. A middle-aged man recovering from myocardial infarction gave a typical response. After matter-of-factly discussing many aspects of his illness and recovery, he began to cry and say, "I never knew anyone cared about me. I just never knew." Then he said, "Men are not supposed to be concerned about such things."

Another response, given by 26% of the total number of patients interviewed, concerned greater realism about the attitudes of others toward them, and a greater feeling of independence accompanying the shattering of some illusions about relationships. A woman who had fractured her hip when she fell on the ice on her way to work after a snowstorm gave a typical response: "My employer was just concerned about the money. From now on I'm going to be more concerned about myself, and what is safe for me to do, and not so dedicated to my job."

General recovery responses

In responding to the general question "What else would you like to tell me about your recovery?" many patients brought up survivor themes. Since the question was very open, responses were especially spontaneous. The similarity of responses is, therefore, interesting.

Almost all psychiatric and alcoholic patients (97%) mentioned stigma in various contexts as an overriding concern. Most frequently mentioned were attitudes of staff and concerns about returning to the community. Typical comments were:

The worst possible thing is being looked down on. I don't feel looked down on by people here, but on the outside it's different.

The hardest problem I have is figuring out what to tell people about where I've been. If I tell the truth I'll have trouble getting a job.

No medical–surgical patients mentioned stigma.

Guilt was expressed by many patients. Medical–surgical patients (34%) whose lifestyle was considered related to their illnesses frequently expressed guilt over being sick. For example, patients with myocardial infarction often mentioned that they had worked too hard, smoked too much, and followed diets that had predisposed them to coronary artery disease. In some instances these patients stated that they knew they were really able to prevent future heart attacks, since now they knew how to alter their lifestyles. This view fails to consider the fact that that no one is in charge of his or her own lifespan and that, while lifestyle is a casual factor, other factors are involved, such as heredity. A typical response of these patients was, "I brought this on myself. I always brought work home from the office. I put everything into my work. I didn't have much time for my family, and I put on weight and smoked a lot."

Most psychiatric and alcoholic patients (90%) expressed a great deal of guilt about their illnesses. Many blamed themselves for their conditions and for not seeking help sooner; they felt they had harmed their families, especially their children. Typical comments were, "My kids have really suffered because of me" and "I should have known to come here sooner, but I tried to tough it out."

Some medical–surgical patients (21%) brought up issues of privacy and intrusion, although only 2 of these patients stated that lack of privacy was avoidable. The others spoke of it as an unpleasant necessity related to their illness. Psychiatric and alcoholic patients spoke of privacy in relation to stigma. Eighty–one percent of psychiatric patients mentioned concern about having to discuss private affairs and wondered about confidentiality. Half of the psychiatric patients mentioned a need for more personal time for reflection apart from the patient group.

While many (86%) psychiatric and alcoholic patients spontaneously mentioned feeling angry, no medical–surgical patients expressed having this feeling. Psychiatric and alcoholic patients mentioned anger as an important aspect of their recovery process—anger at themselves for not seeking help sooner and anger at family and employers for not offering more help and understanding. Several alcoholic patients mentioned that they drank excessively to avoid anger and that without alcohol they were experiencing a great deal of anger.

A heightened awareness of the beauty of nature was brought up by many medical–surgical patients (55%) with a sense of wonder and surprise. In all instances these were patients who had also spoken of a sharper sense of their own mortality as a result of the illness experience. The similarity of responses concerning beauty among these patients was striking, since the interview contained no question about this. Typical comments were:

> Last night I looked out my window at the moon, and I never saw it so beautiful.

> The grass and flowers are so beautiful.

> I just took all this for granted. It is like being made to see with new eyes.

No alcoholic patients gave this response, and very few psychiatric patients made any comment about heightened appreciation of nature (.09%). Those who did speak of it did not emphasize it.

Recovery

In response to the question "What do you do to help yourself recover?" almost all psychiatric and alcoholic patients (90%) described themselves as primary agents of their own recovery. In contrast, many medical–surgical patients (89%) seemed surprised by this question, and were very hesitant before making any response. Their most typical initial response was, "I'm doing what the staff tell me to do." Some medical–surgical patients, however, spoke without hesitation of their own roles in recovery (11%), mentioning learning self-care and participating in various therapies. While the type of illness and treatment is undoubtedly partly responsible for this marked difference in responses of medical–surgical versus psychiatric and alcoholic patients, there are implications for nursing that will be discussed in Chapter 5.

Psychiatric patients emphasized the value of activities in helping them recover, as well as the usefulness of individual and group therapy. Frequently mentioned activities that were viewed by patients as therapeutic were walking, sports, gardening, and painting. Psychiatric and alcoholic patients stressed the valuable role that other patients played in their recovery, by providing companionship and by helping them understand both how others perceive them and the importance of some time alone for reflection.

Medical–surgical patients spoke of helping themselves by walking, eating therapeutic diets, performing therapeutic exercises, and learning self-care. Medical–surgical patients discussed various activities, such as handicrafts more in the context of alleviating boredom than in therapeutic terms.

In response to the question "What do nurses and other staff do that helps you recover?" almost all medical–surgical patients spoke first of cheerfulness and good humor (95%). The second most frequent response involved caring. Typical responses were:

If the nurse comes in with a smile, that just means everything in helping me get better.

Most of these nurses really care. I feel cared about, and not
like a number or a case.

The third most frequent response among medical–surgical
patients had to do with knowledge and skill. A typical response was, "These nurses are specially trained to know
what to look for and what to do."

Psychiatric and alcoholic patients had somewhat different responses to this question. Their first response usually
had to do with avoidance of stigma. Ninety-three percent of
psychiatric and alcoholic patients brought up this concern
in relation to staff. Typical answers were, "They don't talk
down and make us ashamed" and "They don't act like we're
the scum of the earth." The second most frequent response
among psychiatric and alcoholic patients concerned knowledge and skill. Eighty-three percent of these patients spoke
of the importance of nurses' knowledge and skill. A typical
comment was, "They know what our treatment is all about
and they are part of our group program."

An abrupt decrease in contact with health professionals
after the acute phase of illness was over was mentioned by
80% of all patients in the study. Most of these patients
stated that they missed the contact.

Responses to the questions, "Are there things that you
do, that you notice hinder your recovery?" and "Do nurses
and other staff do things that hinder your recovery?" were
minimal among all patients. Frequently they did not respond at all, and when the questions were repeated, most
patients said such things as, "I haven't had any bad experiences" or "I really can't answer that." Probably the facts that
the interviewer had only one contact with patients, that they
were still hospitalized, and that the interviews were taped

affected the responses. Among the few answers other than those cited above were:

> It is important not to put very sick patients in the same room with recovering patients. [medical–surgical]

> Noise is a big problem—I can't rest. [medical–surgical]

> Sometimes we get wakened when it isn't necessary. [medical–surgical]

> Sometimes nurses are grumpy, and that makes it hard on me. [psychiatric]

> It is important not to give a lot of orders. Alcoholic patients find that hard to take.

> One nurse came in and used equipment which was intended for us patients. [psychiatric]

Only .09% of all patients gave substantive response to these questions. The others stated they had had only positive experiences.

Chapter 4

Study of Survivors
of Serious Illness:
Excerpts from
Patient Interviews

The following are excerpts from patients' conversations.
While the comments are preserved, care has been taken to
remove any identifying information.

Patient Recovering from
Acute Depression

What is most important to me now is to have a week to
myself. Just to have time to myself, to do what I want.
There's no way to have that when you have children, and I
have three. I'm waiting for the day when I can have some
time to myself. My husband is away a lot. He used to manage
things, but now I have to manage the money, the kids. I
have so much more responsibility now. Everything and
everyone seems to depend on me. I wonder what to tell
people about why I am here. I'm proud to be here, but I
know many people wouldn't see it that way. What's most
important to me now is my children and my husband. I
don't care so much as I used to about what others think and
want me to do. Like neighbors and friends. I want to get our

family on an even keel. I used to spend a lot of enery trying to please everybody. Now I'm figuring out what's most important to me. I'm thinking about it a lot. I was involved in too many things. I could never say "No." Now I realize I have to have time for myself and I want more time and energy with my family, especially my children. Having to come here really shook me up. It made me see things in a new light, just knowing I really had to come here. What helps me a lot is doing hand work. Knitting, crocheting. It calms me. I like to go out for walks and to the gym. I get a lot out of the group meetings, too, but I need time alone, time to think and try to sort things out.

Patient Recovering from Myocardial Infarction

This comes as a real setback. I just retired. I never could relax before. Always on the go. Well, now I have to relax. My wife and I have been looking forward to this retirement. I'm wondering now if it will all work out, how much time I have left. It's giving me a lot to think about—about what's most important to me. Time to enjoy life with my wife, and time to see my children and grandchildren are most important to me now.

Patient Recovering from Myocardial Infarction

I'm trapped. I feel as though I'm on a suicide mission. My job is full of presseure. I can't give it up. I've got four kids. I'm so caught up in my work. Even my heart attack had to wait half an hour while I finished up some work. I knew I was having the attack but I made myself hang on to finish what I had to do at work. While I was riding here in the

ambulance I kept thinking of my work—of things I still
needed to do. It was only later I began to think of my kids.
But now as I lie here I am thinking of my kids more and I
am beginning to put them first. What the staff do that is
most helpful is helping me stop smoking. I need to stop.
What's least helpful is waking me when it's not necessary.
I've had one attack before this one. I can't seem to change
even though I know the way I work will probably land me in
here again.

Patient Recovering from
Acute Anxiety State

What's most important to me now is keeping the family together. I want to go home to my family. I've been in the
middle of trying to solve everyone else's problems: neighbors, relatives, everyone. I'm smack in the middle. I haven't
been taking care of myself as a person. I have a job, I'm a
wife and a mother, but I'm not taking care of myself. Yester-
day I called my father. He said to me for the first time "I
love you." He's concerned about me. He has helped me
when I needed help. We never talked to each other like that
before. I'm helping myself by relaxing, by taking time for
myself. I play with my hair. I choose what color lipstick to
wear. I can wash my face as often as I want. At home I've
not time, except for a quick shower. At home everyone's life
is in my pocketbook. A key to be made, a watch to be fixed, a
prescription to fill. Errands for everybody. It is so nice now
to be able to look in my purse and find my own lipstick.
Sometimes you have to get in a car accident or burn your
hand or something to stop yourself. I stopped because I just
couldn't manage anymore. I feel much closer to people than
I ever have before. I've been comforted by the other patients
and I comfort them when they need it. The staff seem to

manage to have time whenever anyone is upset. They never talk down to us or act as though we're no good. That means so much.

Patient Recovering from Bleeding Peptic Ulcer

I am a deeply religious person and my illness has made me more religious. I've had to lean on my religion. Illness has crystallized my faith. I had stomach surgery several years ago. That made a big difference in my life. Before that, I had no faith. But in that crisis I turned to God and that made a profound difference in my life. During my first hospitalization I didn't trust anyone on the staff. I felt afraid. Now I feel very confident in the staff and I know that helps me get better. This time I came here for [gastrointestinal] bleeding. They were ready to operate on me. I was bleeding so much. But I prayed, and I asked them to look [gastroscope] one more time and they did. The bleeding had stopped. I didn't need the surgery.

After my first hospitalization I took a step down in my job. I gave it a lot of thought first. I realized I was under too much pressure in my job. I was irritable with my family and I didn't have enough time with them, and then I got sick. I've never regretted changing my job, even though it meant giving up future promotions. We live well enough, and health has become more important to me than material things.

Patient Recovering from Abdominal Surgery

I feel much more concerned with my surroundings than I usually do. I notice more that things are neat and clean. I was really glad for the companionship of the patient across the hall. Our surgery was at about the same time. But other than talking with her I like to keep to myself just now. The nurses have been helpful. I've noticed a change in my reactions toward them. When I was feeling very sick right after my surgery I thought of them as very power-ful—sort of larger than life. Today when I looked at them I suddenly realized they are fallible young women, doing their work.

Patient Recovering from
Acute Depression

I kept digging myself farther and farther away from others. I have three children. I was either drunk or high all the time and I was hurting my children so much because of that. Then one day I stood in the street trying to get run over. Then I got a gun and that got attention. I needed someone to stop me. I keep active here and that helps me get better. I join in the sports program and the group discussions. I wish I had come here four years ago. If it weren't for my kids I wouldn't be getting help now. I really want to go back to them. Even when staff don't have time, they make time to help me when I'm upset. And we patients help each other. I'm afraid to leave here, but still I want to go home. Nobody here treats us like dirt. Nobody puts us down.

Patient Recovering from
Cholecystectomy

What I had seems minor I guess. But it has made a big change in my life. I'm young, I've been very healthy. Very busy with my work. I sort of lost touch with my family. But when I found out I had to have surgery, I phoned my par-ents. They were so concerned and I was so glad to talk with them. And my brother has been visiting me every day. He and I are really growing quite close. It has opened my eyes to be here and to see what can happen to people. I feel much more involved with the people here on this floor than I ever would have thought. I've really changed just since coming here. But I never expected anyone to ask me about it, and it hasn't occurred to me to wonder if other people might feel this way, too. It's as though I've suddenly grown up and become aware of a whole side of life I never knew was there. Like I wouldn't ordinarily talk with an older person, or a black person, or someone very sick. I just kept to my own group of young friends. Here, the differences in age and race and things like that don't seem to be barriers. We're all in the same boat, trying to get well.

Patient Recovering from Hysterectomy

This has been really a routine thing. It hasn't changed anything. We don't want more children (we have two already) and my doctor told me it won't affect my sex life. Nothing has changed for me. I have a part-time job which doesn't interfere with family life. I'll be glad to get home and start doing the things I used to again.

Patient Recovering from Radical Mastectomy

I felt so upset about this operation. I didn't want to have it, and was very depressed. The first room I was in was so dingy. This room is beautiful and that helps my spirits. What made me feel better was helping my roommate. It helped me to be able to help her. I pulled myself together. Then the last few days—I don't know how to tell you. I was looking out the window last night. I never saw the moon so beautiful. It was vivid to me somehow in a way I had never felt before. I felt more alive, more a part of things than I ever have. I guess I'd call it seeing with new eyes.

Patient Recovering from Severe Fractures Caused by Auto Accident

I had an appointment and I kept it even though it was a very rainy day. From now on I'm going to give more thought to what kind of weather it is. I really didn't have to keep that appointment that day. I just always figured nothing would ever happen to me. Now I look at life as a gift. Before, I took it for granted. It could be taken away from me any time. I feel a lot more sympathetic to others. I look at them and see so many who are so sick. I guess being young and healthy I just never thought about this side of life. I feel much more purpose in my life now. I want to be a better husband and father. My religion is a lot stronger. Having the accident makes me realize I have a new opportunity. What helps me is getting up and beginning to do things for myself, and getting out of my room to talk with other patients.

Patient Recovering from Pneumonia

I was so depressed at being here, the bottom dropped out of everything. I'm having to find the inner resources to deal with it. I just can't let myself get down that far again. Surgery attracts people to you—there's the recovery room, the various routines. But I just felt abandoned. I'm starting to feel better. The main thing for me is to find the strength to get over the blues and to be able to take care of myself at home.

Patient Recovering from
Myocardial Infarction

At my age it's time to take it easier. I've got to slow down
a bit. I never acknowledged that—it was always push,
push. I'm going to have to slow down in my business. This
time I'm here for a visit—it was just a visit. I hope I have
more time left. There are things I want to do. I'm having
to think a lot about what's most important to me. The
main thing is my health, and I just never recognized that
before, and I guess I never recognized normal limits. Now
I know my body has its limits to what it can take. I can't
push on no matter how exhausted I am. Maybe I'm just
starting to learn some things I should have learned a lot
earlier. I help myself by doing what the doctors and
nurses tell me to do.

Patient Recovering from
Abdominal Surgery

It made me appreciate a lot of things: the outside, the fresh
air, the grass. I used to take it all for granted. I was on the
verge of death. I came through with dialysis. What I used to
take for granted, I no longer do. It was a shock to my family.
We've all become a lot closer.

Patient Recovering from
Cerebrovascular Accident

I'm glad I worked hard when I was young. I couldn't do it
anymore. This was a warning and I know it. It means I can't
keep pushing myself with working twelve hours every day.
I've made up my mind I'm going to lick this. I don't give in.
But I have to live differently now, and I still haven't figured
out how that will be. I've been thinking maybe I didn't *have*

to push so hard, but I never thought of that before this happened. My wife used to tell me, but I never listened. Now I have to listen.

Patient Recovering from Radical Mastectomy

Something like this gets you down to basics. When I woke up after the surgery I felt the shock of knowing my breast was gone. It was a real hard shock. It takes down the barriers between people. I feel a lot closer to my family. I think sometimes we took each other for granted. I feel a lot better when I go down to the dining room. I can see other people and talk.

Patient Recovering from Myocardial Infarction

What helps me most is knowing the nurses really care about me. It's not just a job to them. The noise is a hindrance to recovery. It's not too quiet. It helps me to talk with my roommate. He and I cheer each other up and give each other a lot of companionship. I'm in a healing period. It's difficult because I'm bored. I've had lots of time to think things over. Being with my family has become very important to me. My business life has been very active—on the train by 7 A.M., home by 5 P.M. Out to dinner several times a week. I was going to retire in two years but now I'm thinking of retiring earlier. I've been on a constant merry-go-round. Perhaps if I had slowed down this would not have happened. The doctor really levels with me and that helps a lot. I know where I stand. This morning I slept until 8 o'clock. I never could sleep after six in the morning. I'm starting to relax. It's going to be hard for me, though, once I go home, to take it easy. The shock of this experience is going to help me. I won't be able to forget this in a hurry.

Patient Recovering from Severe Fracture of Leg After Accident

At first the doctor said I probably would never walk again. That shook me up. Now I'm getting better and I'm thinking things over a lot. I've been very wrapped up in my work. I've gotten a lot out of it but I've also missed a lot. I want to push less and enjoy my life more. I can still remember the doctor saying I might not walk again. It was like a red flag going up and making me stop and think what I'm doing with my life. Being in the hospital has been a real experience. I've met people I'd never have known otherwise. A lot of them are worse off than I am and I've gotten more. . . I guess I'd say more human, from going through this. Our family had a rift, and that is changing since my accident. I hardly ever saw my sister and brother but once this happened they were on the phone long distance every other day. I think sometimes a shock like this can bring families closer together. I think we're going to mend our rift. I hope so.

Patient Recovering from Acute Depression

I never used to be aware of people around me—how they might feel or what they might be going through. I just went along day after day, sort of just making it. Only I didn't realize that then. I wasn't really aware of my kids, either, and of how I was hurting them, being all closed into myself. Now I notice a lot more about other people. And here, I get involved in helping others who are upset. And I've been helped a lot, too, by other patients and by staff. The most important thing for me now is to get home and to be with my children and to be a real parent to them. I know it won't be easy. We've got a lot to work out. They are waiting for me and that means so much. I wonder that I never saw these things before. I've only been here two weeks, but the shock of having to come has really made me see things in a new light. I guess I should have seen this coming, but I didn't. I don't feel ashamed of being here, and it helps that the staff respect the patients.

Patient with Alcoholism, Recovering from Acute Alcoholic Intoxication

When they brought me here I had nothing to say about it. I was on a stretcher. Out cold. I would never have come on my own. But now that I'm here, I'm glad I'm here. I haven't felt so well in years as I do right now. I have an appetite, I sleep, I'm not feeling as though I'll explode if I don't have a drink. Well, I'll be here several weeks, and then I'll be on an outpatient program for a long time. Staff here really know their business. There's no sentimentality, no sermons. We're expected to begin solving our problems with the drinking. I'm part of a group, and we're all struggling with the problem. We have a lot of group discussions, and there's a lot of frankness. I guess by the time we get here, the social cover-ups have been blown. I covered up for years, but now it's out in the open. I can't tell you what a relief that is. I was surprised to find that my family and my boss want to help me, and that they really had pretty good clues to what was going on for a while before I came here. It never occurred to me I'd get any help. It was a process of "hide" and then patch myself up to try to look good. When I came here I had really hit bottom. I was dead drunk and that was all. I suppose a few more bouts like that and I could have killed myself with the stuff. I always minimized the problem, but once I came here in that condition I had to face it and I've got time now to think over a lot of things I've avoided. Like what this is doing to my family and to my work. Having a drink seemed the main thing before, and now I realize how much of my life I've been missing. My kids are growing up, and I'm not getting any younger. I just feel I've got to stick with this treatment program no matter what. What helps me the most is the staff—they are cheerful and human, but they don't fool around. Everyone has to toe the line—getting up for breakfast, going to group meetings, eating right. The other patients help me a lot.

Patient Recovering from Myocardial Infarction

I really did this to myself. I smoked three packs a day. I was under pressure and overweight. I never paid attention to all this health education stuff. Now I figure, if I learn all that they're teaching me, I'll know how to avoid attacks. I think I can prevent it from happening again. I feel that my life can go on just as before.

Patient Recovering from Acute Anxiety State

What helps me most is doing my work. I write and I also do some painting. The staff here are really very good about arranging for me to have the time and the privacy to keep on with my work. I find the group meetings also help, but being able to keep on with my work really helps me not to get totally swallowed up in being a patient. I feel I have one foot in my usual life. I know I can still work and that encourages me. The staff here really respect patients. We are not put down or made to feel we aren't worth anything. Once we go home, if we get upset, we can always come back here for a visit. It helps to know that. I find I value myself more, I value my work more, and I definitely value my independence more than before this happened. I'm beginning to notice and care about other people. I'm making some friends here on this unit. When I get out I want to have a place of my own to live. I just hope I can manage to do it. The staff here are beginning to help me and I'll have some days when I can start looking for an apartment before I leave.

Among these patients and many others there was much reflection and awareness that the illness was related to long-term patterns of behavior. Implied in many patients' comments is "Now it's clear to me but it wasn't before." Lack of awareness of the consequences of lifestyle on their health seemed characteristic of many patients. Illness brought them up short, opening for them new perspectives. Whether or not this changed perspective persists, the fact of its occurrence presents an important opportunity for learning. During the recovery phase patients may be especially open to this kind of learning, which can be life-sustaining and even life-saving. We may speculate that for many patients the changes in values are transitory, while for others they may be of long duration. Research into this issue, with longitudinal studies, would be highly desirable. Nevertheless, any experience that can open new perspectives and promote personal growth is worthy of nurses' efforts, at the time, to potentiate growth. Talking about the experience can help patients maximize the learning. The nurse, when listening to patients, can suggest that it may be hard to hang onto some of these views later, when pressures of work and family life build up, and that planning and reflecting now can help him or her during difficult times that may lie ahead. Some patients may be helped by a diary, which they can reread in the future, thus recalling some of the insights experienced during recovery.

In view of the recent emphasis on lifestyle in relation to health maintenance, it is important, when doing an initial assessment of a sick person, to inquire about his or her daily routine and about any major changes and stresses he or she may be experiencing. While this has been advocated for years, nevertheless many patients are treated strictly in relation to their physical illness, without any consideration of life patterns and stresses that may promote illness.

A related issue involves timing of intervention. Many patients lead lives clearly inimical to health; some patients desperately endure symptoms for years before reaching a "breaking point" when help is sought. It is interesting to speculate on the factors that may be responsible: denial of the seriousness of symptoms; fear of what may be found if health assessment is done; concerns about stigma (particularly for psychiatric patients); worries about financing health care; or lack of awareness of what health care is available. Many patients in the study were clearly in need of intervention much earlier than they received it, which may lead one to question the adequacy of even "good" health check-ups, which focus largely on physical examinations and laboratory data, and minimize the importance of health habits. It is sometimes difficult for patients to ask for help with vague feelings of uneasiness, fatigue, and overreaction to stressful situations. It may be that patients continue in such a state until a clear emergency mandates professional help. Most of the patients in this study who were admitted for medical and psychiatric emergencies, described, in retrospect, that it was clear to them that "something had to happen." To what extent do industrial health programs assist employees to note and act upon warning signals? How free does a client feel simply to go to a health care facility saying, "I don't feel well"? Is the expectation in such facilities that a clear illness must be present to warrant consideration? And in the absence of a clearly identifiable illness, how much assessment is done of the individual's health maintenance habits? How many women, for example, feel that they are "carrying the family in my pocketbook"? How many feel no let-up from the ceaseless work and social pressures that have enveloped their lives? What role can nurses play in earlier detection of illness for individuals? Perhaps an important aspect of nurses' help involves supplementing the medical emphasis on demonstrable pathophysiology with a focus broad enough to include lifestyle. Certainly, once a patient has been admitted to a hospital, nurses can assess lifestyle and stresses and their possible relation to the current illness.

Chapter 5

Study of Survivors of Serious Illness: Implications for Nursing

Introduction

In our emphasis on relieving suffering we may underestimate the personal growth potential that may accompany survival of serious illness. In view of the proliferation of various programs to enhance personal growth, it is ironic that relatively little attention is given to the personal growth possibilities of experiences with serious illness. Nursing's emphasis is necessarily on prevention of illness, relief of distress, and maintenance of health and comfort. The result of this emphasis is that our attention to the personal growth that may accompany illness may be lessened. Unlike such experiences as taking part in an encounter group, illness is not arranged but occurs naturally in the course of living. With their focus on supporting patients during their experiences of serious illness, nurses are in a position to help clients maximize personal growth through their survival. Taking this view also helps the nurse to individualize patient care. For example, when planning care for a patient with radical mastectomy, rather than limiting rehabilitation plans to such usual considerations as exercises and prostheses (important as these are), consideration can be given to both ascertaining the patient's individual responses to the experience and to those factors common to all patients who have this kind of surgery.

Nurses are available to patients in the period just prior to discharge from the hospital, before the resumption of work and family responsibilities. This period, after the acute crisis but before resuming life outside the hospital, may be a very useful one, when values, goals, and future directions can be explored with the patient, and when support can be given to personal growth.

Because of nursing's emphasis on precisely stated objectives and measurable outcomes, it may be difficult for the nurse to deal with less tangible considerations. Personal growth emerging from an encounter with serious illness is more elusive and more variable, for the nurse as well as the patient, than performance of a prescribed exercise. Nevertheless, such questions as, "Survival for what?" and "Where do I go from here?" influence recovery, and have been intuitively acknowledged by skilled nurses. Placing this intuitive understanding within a conceptual framework that draws on the work of theorists concerned with survival can enhance the nursing process. It can sensitize nurses to survival themes in the communications of recovering patients, thus enabling nurses to recognize and support personal growth, and to recognize negative survival patterns as well, so that the nurses, or other health care professionals, may help the patient.

While emphasis on specificity of goals and outcomes is important and necessary, it is also true that some goals are best achieved, not by dogged insistence on and efforts at control, but by letting go, freeing one's attention, allowing things to happen, and allowing oneself to notice what is happening. In the process of carrying out many aspects of care, the nurse can give the recovering patient opportunities to express existential concerns.

Teaching patients individually and in groups provides an opportunity for the nurse to help the patient place the illness experience within the context of his or her daily life, and of his or her values and goals. How often, however, do we who conduct teaching sessions among patients who have had a serious illness, such as myocardial infarction, stress facts about the condition, self-care, and prevention, but leave unasked such questions as, "What was the experience like for you?" and "What is most important to you now?" Teaching patients about their illness is far from being entirely a didactic process during which the nurse imparts facts and skills. Rather, it is a process in which the patient weaves these facts and skills into the fabric of his or her life in light of his or her own values and goals. If the patient is in the process of changing values and goals, the teaching process will be successful to the extent that such changes are considered, and the instruction adapted accordingly.

Hannah Brown* had a myocardial infarction at age 54. She had been an active parent and homemaker. At the time of her illness, her youngest child was finishing high school, two of her other children commuted to college, and a fourth had a job. Her husband was employed as an engineer. Hannah described herself as constantly on the go, whether with shopping, baking, or social activities. She had enjoyed excellent health and the attack came as a shock to her and her family. As she began to recover, Hannah learned a lot about the functioning of the heart and ways to decrease risk factors. She listened as her cardiologist explained that she could resume her life where she left off, with some modifications, particularly in relation to getting more rest, losing some weight, and beginning a program of regular exercise.

As she recovered, Hannah had a great deal of time to reflect on her experience. At first she was preoccupied with

*All names and other identifying information have been changed to protect confidentiality.

gratitude at being alive and sometimes she relived the fear and pain she had gone through. Gradually these concerns lessened and she began to think, "Well, I didn't die. I'm still here. So now what?" She became more aware of the fact that she had passed 50 and she became quietly aware of the fact that she would die someday. Her life had a time limit, and this was something she had not acknowledged before. As she listened to her physician, her husband, and children reassuring her that she could resume her usual life activities after a period of rest, she began to question whether the concerns and activities in which she had previously engaged were really important to her now. She took a fresh look at her children and realized they had grown up. It wasn't really necessary for her to continue doing their laundry, shopping, and errands as she had done. Her volunteer activities in the community no longer held her attention. She began to want to do something she at first thought was idiotic. She wanted to paint. Prior to her marriage, Hannah had done commercial art work and had greatly enjoyed it.

One day, after hearing many reassurances from her nurses and her physician about how she could function largely as she had before, Hannah began to cry. Her nurse was surprised, as recovery was going smoothly, but she listened as Hannah said,

Maybe I don't *want* to do just as I did before. Everyone seems to have plans worked out for me. But I've been through a lot, and I've been thinking about how I want to spend the rest of my life. And I think—I just wonder—if I could do anything in art again. My family doesn't need me to fill the exact same niche I was in. They want me to, but it doesn't have to be that way.

In this situation the nurse was able to work with Hannah and her family, facilitating discussion of these concerns while Hannah was recovering in the hospital. The nurse recognized that these matters affected not only the patient but the family as well, and that failure to consider Hannah's views and goals was leading her to feel isolated and somewhat coerced (through kindly reassurance) to resume her usual activities in the accustomed way.

Reinforcing and Strengthening Personal Growth

The personal growth that may occur as a result of illness can be fostered by listening for survivor themes and recognizing their significance. The nurse can say, for example, "Tell me more about that" or "Give me an example of what you mean" in response to a patient's comment that things are going to be different for him or her from now on. Such interventions need not be lengthy and can occur in the course of carrying out varied nursing functions. The alertness and sensitivity of the nurse to a process of growth and change which may be underway are essential to seeking ways to support and strengthen this process.

This aspect of work with patients rests heavily on values, and it is important for the nurse to be aware of his or her own values, and to realize that these may not coincide with those of the patient. The patient who responds to the illness experience with renewed resolve both to control the events of his or her life and, in essence, to try harder to stay well, may evoke the nurse's admiration more than the patient who speaks of relaxing more and learning to "roll with the punches." On the other hand, the opposite may be true. While recognizing and respecting differences in values, the nurse can raise questions when the patient shows misunderstanding, and can help him or her develop a more realistic assessment of his or her situation. For instance, some medical–surgical patients in this study expressed denial indirectly by discussing their great good fortune compared with that of other patients. This response was most frequent among patients who had been the sickest. A helpful comment might be "Yes, you are lucky to be getting better, but let's talk about ways that you can help yourself stay well." In their emphasis on how much better off they were than others, these patients indicated much denial of what had happened to them and a sense that everything was a matter of luck. They may also have been experiencing a sense of relief just to be alive.

In contrast, some medical–surgical patients in the study spoke as though convinced that as a result of the instruction they were now totally in control of their own lifespan. Such awesome responsibility is not only unrealistic but burdensome and anxiety-laden, and may even precipitate another episode of illness. It is important to examine instruction given to patients to determine whether unrealistic expectations are being fostered. Programs for the education of patients with coronary artery disease may be especially likely to present this difficulty.

Patients whose lifestyle is clearly inimical to their recovery, and who are unable to change the values and priorities that underlie this lifestyle, present a particular challenge to nurses. Because of nurses' broad focus on the patient's responses, rather than the more narrow focus on diagnosis and treatment, nurses may be the first to recognize this problem and its serious implications for recovery. However, referral for personal counseling frequently does not receive high priority in a treatment setting where the emphasis is on care of physical illness. Nurses' recognition of the need for counseling and collaboration with other health professionals to provide this opportunity can be lifesaving.

In addition to counseling, such patients can benefit simply from the empathic presence of the nurse. Nonverbal communication of support and concern can help patients to realize that someone cares about them, and thus may help them to care more about themselves. Patients who are harming themselves by clearly undermining their own health may especially need the nurse's concerned presence. An attitude of openness to patients' and families' concerns is an important aspect of the empathic presence.

Illness presents an opportunity to be and to feel cared for and cared about. Several patients poignantly described this as a new experience for them ("I just never knew anyone cared"). It is an indication of personal growth that these patients could perceive caring and could respond to it. Clearly, these patients were revising their attitudes toward others, based on the realization that others cared for them. It is easy to forget, when working on a busy hospital unit, that some patients, however poised or socially successful they may seem, have lacked human warmth and closeness. For such people, illness carries not only threat and opportunity for fear, but also an opportunity for the demonstration of caring and for developing trust.

The issue of trust comes to the fore because of the patient's relative helplessness. He or she has to depend on others in a way that may not have been necessary since childhood. When others are dependable and show caring, this may help the patient not only in the immediate situation, but also in future relationships. Answering the call bell promptly, being alert and responsive to the patient's physical and emotional needs. and showing that the patient is viewed as an individual are all ways of fostering trust.

Much has been written about the nurse's role in helping patients move through denial to acceptance of illness and to acceptance of the reality of death as a factor in personal growth. It is important to listen for this concern, especially in patients among whom it is likely to be missed—routine surgical patients, for example. The importance of helping patients to deal with denial is often stressed in relation to learning self-care. In addition to this important consideration it is useful to recognize that denial of the serious-

ness of illness and of the possibility of death interferes with
the personal growth that may result from experiencing serious illness. The nurse who helps patients progress through
the denial phase may not only assist them to take responsibility for their own care, but may also help them to open up
significant growth experiences. The clearer and sharper
sense of values and priorities based on the recognition that
life is not endless and a heightened sense of beauty, with its
opportunities for self-healing and enjoyment, are examples.

Of course, not all change is positive. The literature
points out such negative changes as constriction of interests
and psychic numbing as examples of negative outcomes of
survivor experiences. Patients in this study, when asked
about changes, mentioned positive changes. Possibly some
negative changes, such as apathy, may become evident later
to these patients, or to the patients' close associates. Some
patients may have been aware of negative changes at the
time of the interview but had decided not to mention them.
Subsequent interviews with the same patient might have
elicited this information.

Depression, apathy, withdrawal, and unfocused hyper-
activity are all examples of outcomes that may present difficulties with work and home life. While such difficulties
are often recognized by the patient and by others, they
may not be viewed as common responses among survivors,
but rather as an individual's failure to measure up to expectations. When the patient and those caring for him or
her view these negative outcomes within the context of a
survivor experience, greater patience may be extended and
further efforts may be made by the patient and others to
help him or her move through these crippling manifesta-
tions of survivorhood to more positive outcomes. The expectations of patients for themselves, and of families and
especially of health care professionals for them, are often

patently unrealistic, and may serve to develop a sense of failure or mystification among patients. Thus expectations that patients will move through catastrophic experiences, such as strokes, without overt expressions of anger, that those with significant losses, such as experienced by mastectomy patients, will "accept" this change within the week or two of hospitalization are at variance with knowledge about human responses. One woman in the study who had had a hysterectomy mentioned that she cried, but was puzzled by the tears. The surgery was presented to her as routine and unlikely to affect her future life in any way, since she was in her forties. Acknowledgment of the loss by the interviewer ("Tears are natural when you have lost something") helped the patient view the tears not as mysterious and inappropriate, but as an understandable human response to a loss.

Use of Groups

While sense of community, concern for others, and interdependence are stressed as part of treatment programs for alcoholic and psychiatric patients, the possibility that physical illness also provides the opportunity to grow in these areas is less often acknowledged.

Greater use of groups as an aspect of therapy among psychiatric and alcoholic patients than among medical–surgical patients is understandable in light of patients conditions and requirements for treatment. While acknowledging these treatment differences, the need of medical–surgical patients to withdraw and to focus upon themselves is emphasized more than development of a greater sense of community and concern for others. Both approaches may be operative to varying degrees.

Patients can benefit from knowing that the experiences they are going through are like those of others in similar circumstances. A comment from the nurse that many people experience similar feelings during illness and recovery can help patients recognize these feelings as part of a human process. Patients can also share their views with one another during group sessions. Although groups in the medical–surgical setting are used primarily for patient teaching, such groups can readily encompass, in addition to teaching, sharing of experiences, feelings and exploration of the effects of the illness experience on values, goals, and future plans.

Group teaching of surgical patients, for instance, can readily provide opportunities for patients to show their concern for one another, to recognize the similarity of many of their anxieties, and to provide peer support in recognizing and coping with such common, but often unexpressed, feelings as anger at having to go through the experience, anger at the pain and at the loss of body parts. Concern about loss of privacy (necessary or unnecessary) and feelings of loss of dignity experienced during various procedures can be shared usefully in patient groups. While, ideally, patients can take the opportunity to deal with these feelings with the support of family, friends, nurses, and personal physician, sometimes such support is limited. Recovery may be made more difficult by feelings of anger and humiliation which the patient finds difficult or impossible to cope with alone. Realizing that such feelings are the natural and often inevitable consequences of illness and surgery, and do not necessarily imply neglect by staff, can help patients express these feelings.

The patients' environment during the recovery phase can foster a heightened sense of community. For example, the availability of a kitchenette gave one woman in the study an opportunity to find a companionship, understanding, and increased recognition of interdependence with another patient that transcended social barriers. Group dining areas and recreation areas provide similar opportunities.

Anger

Although alcoholic and psychiatric patients spoke freely about anger and their efforts to deal with it, no medical–surgical patients described anger as a problem. In view of the interruptions in their lives, losses, and pain experienced, it is likely that medical–surgical patients felt less free to discuss anger than the other patients in the study. While coping with anger is viewed as a legitimate concern in the treatment of psychiatric and alcoholic patients, this aspect of experience may be given less recognition among medical–surgical patients. It is difficult, when one is sick and being cared for, to express the anger that is a natural consequence of the physical and psychological stresses that patients undergo. It is also possible that dealing with anger has become a more accepted part of the professional socialization of psychiatric nurses, although the needs of medical–surgical patients for this aspect of care have been emphasized in the literature. Ann Kliman (1978) has vividly described the frequently unmet psychological needs of medical–surgical patients, among which is the need to recognize and express anger. That unexpressed anger is an important obstacle to recovery has been widely recognized, but application of this concept in the medical–surgical setting should be emphasized. With the skilled assistance of a nurse, individual patients and groups of patients can be supported and helped to recognize anger as an acceptable and natural response to illness. Medical–surgical patients in the study spoke readily about their fears. It may be that expression of this emotion, which can call forth reassurances and explanations from staff, is easier and more acceptable to express in the medical–surgical setting than expression of anger.

Privacy

A few medical–surgical patients stated that they experienced avoidable disregard of their privacy; more of them discussed invasion of privacy as a necessary but unwelcome part of the illness experience. The necessity to protect the patient's privacy has been stressed in nursing literature (Smith 1969; Stillman 1978). Half of the psychiatric patients in the study mentioned a desire for greater privacy from the patient group. They mentioned walks outdoors and opportunities to go to the gym as welcome occasions for some personal privacy and reflection.

While carrying out active, necessary treatment functions, it is easy to forget a patient's need for privacy. Pressure on the nurse is ordinarily in the direction of getting things done for and with the patient. Seldom are there reminders within the work group concerning patients' privacy. When things are getting done, staff's work is also being accomplished, whereas provision of privacy may require some rescheduling of work or reevaluation of priorities.

Although patients indicated that invasions of privacy were, for the most part, unavoidable, it is important to remember how constricted a hospitalized patient's living space is and how important, for this reason, privacy can be. When one has only one drawer or one locker, it becomes especially important to have at least that space to oneself. Patients have few options about the people who will share their living area. Ordinarily such decisions are made by others in the institution for reasons that have little to do with compatibility. Frequently moves to new units are made, requiring adjustment to still other patients and staff and further erosion of privacy.

Appreciation of Nature's Beauty

A heightened appreciation of beauty was frequent among those medical–surgical patients in the study who had experienced a greater sense of their own mortality, although they were not necessarily the sickest patients. Many of them described this experience as a veil being lifted or as seeing with new eyes. They described transforming experiences in which they felt in harmony with nature and, in some instances, merged with nature. Patients described this as a recurring experience and not as a one-time, fleeting perception. Although it is generally agreed that such quickened awareness of beauty is an indication of psychological growth, various authors describe the dynamics differently.

Maslow (1971) describes these as peak experiences and relates them to the psychological growth characteristic of self-actualizing people. Jung (1953) stresses the importance of awareness of one's own future death as central to developing maturity, and describes heightened awareness of beauty in terms of being more in touch with the unconscious. Kübler-Ross (1969) has described the importance of recognizing the reality of death in enriching the quality of life. Whatever its origins, the experience is described as liberating, as a source of healing, and as an enrichment of life. Fostering this experience may thus be viewed as important for those in the helping professions. Acknowledging the reality of death may assist patients toward these subjective experiences of awareness of beauty and closeness to nature, and nurses, through support, can encourage this acknowledgment.

Contact with nature, while considered important in the past (as, for example, in the care of patients with tuberculosis), has received less emphasis recently with the growing stress on drug therapy, surgery, radiation, and the like. However, the importance of environment in the care of the sick is being increasingly recognized. The hazards of cutting individuals off from their usual contact with natural light and a view of the outdoors with its variations of day and night have been extensively written about in relation to the environment of the intensive care unit. Less emphasis has been placed on the patient's environment during recovery from illness. In fact, the drastic shortening of hospitalization in order to contain costs often means that patients are discharged when they are just beginning to recover. Unless careful attention is given to discharge planning and to some professional nursing involvement with initial care at home, it is possible that attention paid to the patient's environment during recovery may be scanty, except in situations in which families are able to provide for this.

Opportunity for contact with nature through windows, and later by being outdoors, may help foster a heightened appreciation of the beauty of nature. The use of a patio or porch area, unfortunately relatively infrequent in many general hospitals, would be highly desirable for recovering patients. After discharge, patients and their families can be encouraged to provide opportunities for them to go outdoors into a garden, to a park, when this is feasible, or for drives. Instruction of patients and families prior to discharge tends to focus on medications to be taken, exercises to be done, and so on, with less emphasis on the environment's importance in fostering recovery.

Self-Help

Many medical–surgical patients in the study viewed themselves as relatively passive during the recovery process. Emphasis was on doing what they were told and following directions. In contrast, most psychiatric and alcoholic patients viewed themselves as active participants in their own recovery. Different conditions and treatment modalities account for much of this difference. Confinement to bed, inability to care for physical needs, and being the recipient of others' ministrations (with little choice being realistically available) make passivity and docility adaptive behavior in a medical–surgical environment. Nevertheless, as patients recover it is possible to stress their responsibility for self-care and to help them view their participation as not merely following orders, but as a way of participating actively in their own recovery. An appropriate environment can foster this participation. A dining area where patients can sit together at tables, lounges with some provisions for recreational activities, and kitchenettes for preparing snacks are examples of facilities that foster participation and self-care but that are unfortunately often unavailable to patients who are recovering in general hospitals.

Stigma

Stigma was a prevalent problem among psychiatric and alcoholic patients in the study. Emphasis on the absence of stigma in supportive therapeutic environments may lead staff to forget that patients do experience stigma, as well as other concerns about condescension, invasion of privacy, and a need to discuss their feelings about stigma. Patients were quick to elaborate on the difference between the staff's view of their conditions and the views of such others as employers, friends, and family. The importance that patients placed upon staff attitudes of acceptance was very pronounced, as was their concern with getting help in dealing with stigmatizing attitudes of those outside the hospital.

The difference in responses between medical–surgical patients and psychiatric and alcoholic patients in relation to stigma was marked, and understandable in view of social attitudes. Although alcoholic patients were in a general hospital environment, they mentioned stigma as an important concern; thus, stigma persisted for them, even in a nonstigmatizing setting. The data emphasize the extent to which the burden of stigma attaches to and complicates the recovery of psychiatric and alcoholic patients, in contrast to medical–surgical patients. It is interesting to consider that, although medical–surgical patients are not free of self-destructive behavior (excessively long hours of work, overeating and injudicious eating patterns, excessive smoking, and so on,), these patients did not bring up the problem of stigma, although they did mention guilt. It is likely that society's attitudes are more accepting of some forms of self-destructiveness than of others, thus sparing the hard-driving worker with a bleeding peptic ulcer from the stigma that attaches to a patient hospitalized for depression.

Patients' Perceptions of What Helps Them Recover

Medical–surgical patients, particularly, emphasized the importance of the nurses' moods to their recovery. With the necessary emphasis on specific nursing interventions, it is possible to overlook the importance to patients of nurses' moods. While no one can be expected to be genuinely cheerful all the time, it is important for nurses to be aware of their moods and to try to avoid exposing patients to moods that may stimulate anxiety and impede recovery. Patients said such things as, "When the nurse came in cranky I could feel myself get nervous, and I wouldn't get over it until another nurse came in who was cheerful." Even though the nurse carries out required care, a mood that conveys irritability and possible unwillingness to care for the

patient can stimulate anxiety and thus interfere with maintenance of the physical and emotional states that are condu-
cive to recovery. Lessening or avoiding contact with a particularly anxious patient when one is irritable or gloomy can
be as necessary as avoiding contact with postoperative patients when one has a cold, assuming, of course, that care
can be provided by other staff temporarily.

The respect for and awareness of nurses' knowledge
and skill, indicated as important by all three categories of
patients in the study, was surprising in view of media ste-
reotypes portraying nurses as mindless appendages to physicians. Although nurses clearly have less power in decision
making than physicians, patients in the study were aware of
the importance of nurses' knowledge and skill, underlined
by the fact that direct care and observation were carried out
largely by nurses over the greater part of the day. Patients'
emphasis on the importance of nurses' knowledge and skill
may indicate that they learned a good deal about what
nurses do during their illness. It may also be related to the
fact that the interviewer was a nurse, and may indicate a
desire to please her.

In describing helpful behavior of nurses, patients discussed occasions when nurses went out of their way to help
them, showed recognition of their individual needs, and
exhibited an attitude of caring. One incident involved a
patient who had packed his belongings and who was sitting
in a wheelchair awaiting transfer to another unit. He waited
for several hours, while various busy nurses came and went.
Then one nurse noticed him as she was going off duty,
inquired about his transfer, and took him to his new unit.
(This incident suggests considerable passivity on the part of
this medical–surgical patient, who did not ask about ar-
rangements for his transfer.)

The emphasis that psychiatric patients gave to such activities as walking, sports, handicrafts, and gardening in

helping their recovery highlights the importance of these activities to patients. Perhaps with the growing recognition of the importance of the nurse's role in therapeutic communication, nurses' appreciation of the value of such activities for patients may be lessened, and should be reemphasized without detracting from the importance of the counseling role. Nurses can stress the need for facilities for such activities, which, in an era of high costs, may be viewed as nonessential.

While acknowledging the many positive responses of patients concerning their care, it seems likely that the dearth of negative comments may be related to patients' feelings of vulnerability in the treatment setting, making tape-recorded comments on this topic too threatening. Had there been continuing interviews with each patient, more negative comments may have been expressed. In light of the many frustrations, discomforts, losses, and disappointments inherent in most illness situations, it is likely that many patients did not feel free to comment on these aspects of their experience.

Because patients' changes in values and priorities inevitably affect their families, and because families may be going through their own reassessment of values and priorities as a result of the illness of a family member, it is important for the nurse to foster communication between patient and family about these matters. In the preoccupation with physical aspects of recovery or possibly in an effort to convey to one another that nothing has changed, these important discussions between patient and family may be delayed. When families are aware of the patient's changing values and view these in light of a long term-treatment program, they may be helped to support him or her in making the necessary changes in lifestyle. Discussing changes in values and their long-term implications with the patient may help families to avoid giving repeated admonitions to follow orders and do what is healthy, which often becomes a source of irritation, and may even impede desirable changes in the patient's behavior. The importance of working with families is underscored by the frequency and intensity with which patients in the study spoke about the importance of family to them. Group discussions that include patient, family, and nurse held prior to discharge from the hospital can facilitate realistic planning for the recovery period as well as discussion of possible changes in goals and priorities.

Chapter 6

Study of Recovery: A Relevant Concept for Nursing Care

Doreen Anne Kolditz
Rose Ann Naughton

Introduction

Observations of patients ready for discharge prompted interest in the process of recovery and led to the study discussed in this chapter. Some patients, when told by their physicians that they were ready for discharge, accepted the decision and went home as planned. Other patients stated that, for a variety of reasons, they did not feel ready for discharge.

Some patients in the former group may have felt ready for discharge, while some may have merely acquiesced to the authority of the physician and returned home as planned. It would be interesting to identify the group who conformed to the physician's decision and see if their time for full recovery was affected or if hospital readmission occurred soon thereafter. However, this would require another study.

An earlier version of this chapter appeared as "Patients' Definitions of Recovery from Acute Illness," in *Clinical Perspectives in Nursing Research*, ed. by M. Janice Nelson, New York: Teachers College Press, 1978.

Of the patients who did not feel ready for discharge, some went home a few days later while others developed symptoms or sustained an accident requiring a continuation of the hospital stay. The question arises as to whether this latter group may have been unconsciously identifying a need for help based upon the frequency and regularity of these occurrences.

The above observations led to two questions: How do patients themselves decide they are ready for discharge? What are the criteria they use?

At present, readiness for discharge is determined primarily by the physician, who bases his judgment on clinical parameters. As hospital costs increase, third-party payers (private and governmental), have exercised greater control on criteria for length of stay in an attempt to decrease hospital costs. Length of stay is classified by diagnosis; that is, a given diagnosis usually requires X number of days hospitalization. Documented justification by the physician is needed if the expected stay is exceeded. Usually social and psychological factors are not considered valid reasons to postpone discharge.

Physician determination and criteria from third-party payers leave little choice or option for the patient. Are patients' criteria for discharge important? Studies have shown that people who have input into decisions are more likely to carry them out. Furthermore, people who set their own goals are more likely to achieve them. These same principles are used to teach those who must learn new health behaviors.

If more were known about patient criteria for discharge, hospital readmissions might be lessened. Some patients might have a hospital course with fewer complications. In the long run, with a better mesh of institutional and patient goals, health care institutions could serve the

public better and satisfy the need to keep the costs at a
reasonable level.

Review of the Literature

A review of the literature revealed little about the process
of recovery, particularly from the patient's point of view.
However, the writings of several authors were helpful in
giving direction to the study. For example, Parsons's
(1972) definition of health and illness was useful in cate-
gorizing patient responses and interpreting the results.
From a sociological perspective, Parsons defines health as
the ability of an individual to carry out roles and tasks for
which he has been socialized. In contrast, illness is defined
as the exemption from and inability to carry out these
roles and tasks.

Other authors cite the influence of sociological variables on definitions of health and illness. Koos (1954) found
that health attitudes and actions are significantly influenced
by the socioeconomic group to which a family belongs.
Saunders (1954), in his study of Mexican Americans in the
southwest, showed that the manner in which illness is
treated and the extent to which services are utilized are
linked to ethnicity. Zborowski (1969) also showed that eth-
nic background influenced responses to pain. Several other
studies also pointed out that such sociological variables as
sex, marital status, age, religion, ethnicity, and socioeconomic status influence the way in which health and illness
are defined.

Since these sociological variables have been seen to
have a strong influence on health and illness attitudes and
behaviors, this study focused on these variables in relation

to how patients define recovery. Although other variables, such as psychological ones, would influence definitions of recovery, they were not considered in this study.

The Study

The process of recovery suggests that a person has been ill and is becoming well again. This study is concerned with factors considered important by patients in determining their readiness for discharge from the hospital. It also addresses itself to factors patients considered important in determining full recovery. Readiness for discharge and factors necessary for full recovery were considered part of the recovery process.

A questionnaire was developed so that patients could weigh the relative importance of certain factors in telling them when they felt ready for discharge and when they felt fully recovered. Content for the questionnaire was developed from patients themselves. They were asked what kinds of things would tell them that they were ready to go home and what factors would tell them they were fully recovered. These factors were then listed and categorized as illustrated in Tables 1 and 2.

The two main categories of cues were internal and external cues. Internal cues were those that emanated from within the patient. These included: physical cues that dealt with pain, wound healing, and the like; feeling tone cues, involving emotional responses such as fear and worry; and capability cues that involved ability for self-care such as walking, dressing, and bathing. External cues were those that came from such others as health care personnel, family, and friends.

Patients were asked to rate each cue as being very important, somewhat important, or not important. Both scales

TABLE 1   Cue Categories in Readiness for Discharge Scale

Internal Cues

Physical Cues
   My wound is healed or almost healed.
   My appetite is getting back to normal.
   I have no pain or only slight pain.
   I'm getting stronger and my energy is increasing.
   My sleeping is getting back to normal.

Feeling Tone Cues
   My spirits are getting back to normal.
   I feel less afraid.
   I feel less worried about being sick.
   I feel less down in the dumps.
   I feel ready to go home.

Capability Cues
   I am able to get around without help.
   I am able to go outside without help.
   I can do things for myself, for instance, wash, walk, dress, etc.
   I have no worries how I'll manage at home.
   I'll be able to do light work around the house, shopping, cooking, etc.

External Cues

Cues from Medical and Nursing Personnel
   My blood pressure and temperature are taken less often.
   I get fewer medicines.
   The doctor tells me I'm ready to go home.
   The nurses tell me I'm ready to do more for myself.
   The doctors and nurses come to see me less often.

Cues from Family and Friends
   My friends and family tell me I'm looking better.
   My friends and family tell me I'm ready to go home.
   My family and friends don't worry about me like they did after the operation.
   Others tell me about the problems at home.
   My family and friends treat me more as usual.

included the same cue categories; the Full Recovery Scale contained 12 items compared with 25 items on the scale for readiness to go home. In addition to the scales shown, patients were asked to identify the most important cue on the readiness scale, the person who was the best judge of their readiness for discharge, and to estimate how long it would be before they felt fully recovered.

TABLE 2   Cue Categories in Full Recovery Scale

Internal Cues

Physical Cues
My pain has disappeared.
My wound is healed.
My sleeping is back to normal.
My appetite is back to normal.
My energy is back to normal.

Feeling Tone Cues
My spirits are back to normal.
I no longer worry about problems with my operation.
I feel fully recovered.

Capability Cues
I'm able to carry out my usual activities, like using public transportation, going to work, driving, shopping, sports, going to meetings, etc.
I'm able to carry out my usual activities, like housework, repairs around the house, hobbies, etc.

External Cues

My doctor says I'm fully recovered.
My family allows me to take on my usual responsibilities.

Two hundred patients were interviewed for the study. The patients were essentially well before hospitalization, had had abdominal surgery for a benign condition, and had had an uncomplicated postoperative course. It was expected that after this illness, the patients would return to their former level of functioning. Patients were interviewed at a point during their hospital stay when they were ambulatory, on a regular diet, and within a few days of discharge.

The sample of 200 patients consisted of 99 women and 101 men who ranged in age from 20 to 70 years. Most patients were American born and married. Sixty-five percent were white, 25% were black and 10% were Hispanic. Three religious faiths—Jewish, Protestant, and Catholic—were evenly distributed. Socioeconomic groupings, as determined by the Hollingshead Two Factor Index (1957) (occupations and education), were represented in all groupings with the exception of the lowest educational category.

Results

Data collected from the patient interviews focuses on the "very important" responses to the various cues. Table 3 shows the rank order of very important responses for all patients for readiness to go home.

The results of the rank order are interesting and quite surprising. If nurses or physicians were asked to rate the same items, their responses would undoubtedly be different. As mentioned previously, physicians base their judgments on such clinical data as status of the wound, laboratory data, and temperature. For patients, items dealing directly with the consequences of surgery, such as wound healing and pain, are ranked 6th and 10th respectively. Perhaps this is because pain and a healing would were to be expected and, therefore, were of lesser importance in determining readiness for discharge. It may also be that patients felt these cues were more the physician's concern than theirs.

The first 11 items represent those cues felt to be very important by over 50% of the sample. Of these 11 cues, only one is classified as external; all other cues are internal. The external cue selected was the physician's judgment of readiness to go home. This was seen as very important by 83% of the subjects. Most patients also rated this as the most important cue on the scale and saw the physician as the best judge of readiness for discharge. These results are not surprising, since the physician is often looked upon as an authoritative and knowledgeable person whose decisions are to be respected and followed.

While the results concerning the ranking of the physician's judgment are not surprising, what is surprising is that this cue was 5 percentage points below the first cue, "I'm getting stronger and my energy is increasing." One might speculate that strength and energy are directly related to the two next-ranked items dealing with the patient's capa-

TABLE 3 Rank Order of "Very Important" Responses to Cues to Readiness for Discharge

Rank	Response	%
1	I'm getting stronger and my energy is increasing.	88
2	I am able to get around without help.	83.5
3.5	I can do things for myself, for instance, wash, walk, dress, etc.	83
3.5	The doctor tells me I'm ready to go home.	83
5	I feel ready to go home.	82.5
6	My wound is healed or almost healed.	71
7	My spirits are getting back to normal.	70
8	I am able to go outside without help.	65
9	I have no worries about how I'll manage at home.	64
10	I have no pain or only slight pain.	59.5
11	I feel less worried about being sick.	57
12	My appetite is getting back to normal.	48
13.5	My blood pressure and temperature are taken less often.	47.5
13.5	I feel less afraid.	47.5
15	My sleeping is getting back to normal.	46
16	The nurses tell me I'm ready to do more for myself.	45.5
17	I get fewer medicines.	44.5
18	I feel less down in the dumps.	44
19	My friends and family tell me I'm looking better.	43
20	My family and friends treat me more as usual.	41.5
21	The doctors and nurses come to see me less often.	40.5
22	My family and friends don't worry about me like they did after the operation.	39.5
23	I'll be able to do light work around the house, shopping, cooking, etc.	36.5
24	My friends and family tell me I'm ready to go home.	26
25	Others tell me about the problems at home.	16

bilities for self-care. It seems obvious that strength and energy are needed to be able to care for oneself.

The strength and energy item may also be classified as a feeling tone cue. As indicated in the rank order, two feeling tone cues ranked within the top 11 very important cues. In interviewing patients for the study, it was apparent that many patients experienced depression following surgery. One woman patient described it as a feeling similar to the postpartum blues and labeled it the "postsurgery blues."

Some patients stated that they cried for no apparent reason. Another patient, on the verge of tears, stated that the nurses could give her something for the pain but couldn't understand how she felt. These feelings were frightening for patients. When one feels depressed and does not understand why, the level of strength and energy and general feeling of well-being are decreased.

The cue "I feel less down in the dumps" ranked 18th. This appears to contradict the speculation that depression is related to energy level. However, many patients felt this was a somewhat negative response and said they never felt "down" or didn't consider it very important. The item "My spirits are getting back to normal" may have related more directly to the feeling of depression, since it was not looked upon as bad or negative. This item was considered to be very important by 70% of the subjects in the study.

In summary, for all subjects in the study the very important cues for readiness to go home included a need for:

1. increased strength and energy
2. the ability to care for oneself
3. the decision of the physician as to readiness for discharge
4. a resolution to the sequelae of the surgery—lessened pain and a healing wound
5. feeling states (spirits) to be returning to normal

Table 4 gives the rank order of very important responses for all patients for full recovery. Over 50% of the patients considered all items as being very important. It is difficult to know if these positive responses truly reflect patients' definitions of full recovery first, because patients were still hospitalized and second because there were only 12 items on this scale, compared with 25 items on the scale for readiness to go home.

TABLE 4 Rank Order of "Very important" Responses to Cues to Full Recovery

Rank	Response	%
1	My energy is back to normal.	89.5
2	I feel fully recovered.	88.5
3	I am able to carry out my usual activities, like using public transportation, going to work, driving, shopping, sports, going to meetings, etc.	86.5
4	My wound is healed.	81.5
5	My pain has disappeared.	79.5
6	I'm able to carry out my usual activities, like housework, repairs around the house, hobbies, etc.	76.5
7	My doctor says I'm fully recovered.	74
8	I no longer worry about problems with my operation.	70
9	My spirits are back to normal.	66
10	My family allows me to take on my usual responsibilities.	62
11	My sleeping is back to normal.	60
12	My appetite is back to normal.	57

Nevertheless, the responses are interesting. Again, energy level ranks number one. Close to it, in second place, is the patient's own estimate of being fully recovered. The physician's judgment of full recovery is ranked 7th. These rank orders are in keeping with the responses to the question of who was the best judge of full recovery, to which 49% of the respondents indicated they were the best judge. It would seem that for these patients, full recovery represents a greater degree of self-determination. The physician, while important, is viewed as far less important in determining whether or not the patient is fully recovered. Perhaps patients were able at this point to project themselves into the future when they would be fully recovered, and when they would be in their own surroundings and thereby have more control over their situations.

The most important cue for full recovery was the ability to carry out usual activities. This response is in keeping with Parsons's (1972) sick role theory and the writings of

Koos (1954). These authors point out that illness is seen as interference with the ability to carry out role responsibilities and the activities of daily living.

The return of strength and energy is ranked number one again, and again raises the question of whether or not energy level is strictly a physical cue. In all probability it also includes feelings of well-being and the ability to cope with life as usual.

Items dealing directly with the surgical event (wound and pain) were not as important to the patients for readiness to return home as other cues were. They were, however, of greater importance in determining full recovery.

Capability cues were ranked high on both scales. The ability to carry on usual responsibilities was considered by patients as the most important cue for full recovery. This tends to support Parsons's sick role definition. If illness is seen as the inability to carry out role and task responsibilities, then wellness, or in this case, recovery becomes the ability to do this.

The importance of feeling tone cues is also evident in the responses on both scales. As was noted previously, many patients interviewed stated they felt dejected and depressed postsurgery. Thus, the role of "spirits" becoming normal were important for recovery.

The Influence of Sociological Variables

As was anticipated, sociological variables did, indeed, influence patient responses.

Socioeconomic status

Socioeconomic status influenced responses more than any other independent variable. This is in keeping with

Kohn's (1969) observation that socioeconomic status has a very strong influence on attitudes and opinions.

Patients in the upper socioeconomic group were very selective in rating items as being very important, rating very few as such. Most valued by this group were items related to their own capabilities and self-reliance. With the exception of the physician, all other responses were not considered very important.

Patients in the lower socioeconomic group indicated many factors as very important. This group tended to place more reliance on physical cues for recovery than did the upper socioeconomic patients.

Ethnic group

White patients' responses, being the majority in the study, paralleled those of the entire group. They rated items very important less frequently, capability cues were preferred more often than physical and feeling tone cues, and external cues were considered to be less important.

Black patients were somewhat similar to white patients in their responses. Blacks also felt capability and physical cues to be very important, but they considered external cues to be more important than did white subjects.

Hispanic subjects showed the most variation in their responses in comparison with the other two groups. They leaned heavily on cues from family and friends and feeling tone cues for determining recovery, and they placed less importance on capability cues.

Religious groups

All religious groups valued capability cues as being very important. Jewish subjects placed much less value on external cues than did the other two religious groups.

Religion and ethnicity variables were influenced by socioeconomic status. For example, Jewish subjects were primarily white and of the upper socioeconomic group. Black subjects were primarily Protestant and of the lower socioeconomic group. When looking at the various responses of the Jewish and black subjects and controlling for socioeconomic status, the influence of socioeconomic status is evident. This finding raises the question of whether nurses can assist patients to broaden their coping skills as an aid to recovery. For example, can patients whose pattern is to rely primarily on the views of others be assisted to take fuller account of their own views?

Sex

Male subjects valued capability cues more frequently than did female subjects. Women, on the other hand, placed greater emphasis on their own feelings and cues from family and friends as determinants for recovery. These results may be due to the different socialization processes for males and females in our society. Men have been taught to be self-reliant and not to show their emotions, while women have been taught to be more emotional and dependent. The results in this study may be different a few years from now with the impact of the women's movement on the socialization process. It may be that nurses can help both men and women during recovery by assisting them to develop aspects of themselves which their socialization has denied.

Age

There was one age group that showed significantly different responses from all other groups: the oldest age group of 61–70 years. They regarded external cues from physicians and nurses as less important than any other group. Furthermore, they saw their own estimation of recovery as being more important than that of the physician. Capability cues were also valued as very important more often for this group. Thus, the older age group could be characterized as strongly emphasizing reliance on self and the ability to care for self as important determinants for recovery.

Fear of loss of independence because of advancing age, combined with an illness that further threatens this loss, may be related to the fact that older people place emphasis on capability cues and their own estimate of recovery. It is essential that caregivers make a particular effort to respect older patients' assessment of their abilities, and to use this assessment in plans that help the older person maintain independence.

Type of Surgery

There were two major differences in responses between the patients having major abdominal surgery and those having hernia repairs. First, those having major abdominal surgery rated all items as very important more frequently. In addition, feeling tone cues and reliance upon the physician were cues rated very important more often by patients with major abdominal surgery than those with hernia repairs. Second, those patients with hernia repairs placed greater importance on the lessening and disappearance of pain.

The reasons for these differences seem apparent and are most probably related to the extent and recency of the surgery. Patients with hernia repairs were interviewed within 1 to 2 days postsurgery. Their concern at that time was with pain. Those with major abdominal surgery were interviewed further along in the postoperative period. Their surgery was more extensive and therefore, they would be likely to place greater reliance on the physician's opinion.

Nursing Implications

In discussing the nursing implications of this study, some of its limitations should be kept in mind. The sample in the study represents one type of illness: abdominal surgery. Nevertheless, it represents a beginning effort to develop a concept of recovery and a preliminary search to understand patient criteria for recovery better. The results of this study have potential for enhancing the care of patients and may also be of assistance in helping spark further research in the area.

As has been seen, patients have their own criteria for recovery. For the most part, these criteria are subjective, and very personal, and differ greatly from those of the physician, whose criteria are based on objective data, observation, and laboratory tests.

The three main areas that patients identified as being very important for recovery were spirits returning to normal, return of strength and energy, and capability. All three areas are probably interrelated. Feelings can influence strength and energy and thus affect the ability to care for oneself.

Patients identifying the importance of spirits returning to normal also described feelings of depression, which they felt to be abnormal. Patients prepared preoperatively for these feelings of depression and lack of strength might be able to cope better. They could then utilize their energies more constructively instead of diverting them toward denying or suppressing these "abnormal" feelings. Helping patients explore and identify their expectations for recovery could help them set realistic, achievable goals. What impact will the surgery have on lifestyle, work, or family relationships? Just what can be expected in relation to the time sequence for the resumption of usual activities?

Postoperatively, the nurse could be of great assistance and comfort to patients by being sensitive to the behavioral cues and feelings being communicated. By skillful use of knowledge from behavioral sciences, the nurse could help the patients gain insight into their behavior and feelings. It is important to note that the nurse should not identify feelings for the patient. The patient should be assisted to identify them himself or herself. Because the insights are the patient's and not someone else's, he or she is able to deal with them better.

Care planned in relation to the patients' energy levels could help them exert more control over their care and thus decrease their sense of helplessness and depression. All too often care is planned around staff needs and goals, leaving little room for individualized care. Again, needs and goals identified by patients are the ones most likely to be met and achieved. Through astute observation of patient behavior and discussion with him or her, nurse and patient could work out a plan of care specific for that patient. This plan would then help the patient test out capabilities at a time when energy level and strength are greatest. The plan would then be used at a time when success is most likely. Successful achievement enhances the patient's sense of self-worth. Pacing activities is very important in order not to deplete strength and energy all at once.

No surgery or patient is "routine." The implications of patient criteria for recovery require skill and creativity on the part of the nurse. Working with patients and their concerns results in better care for patients and better use of the nurse's expertise.

Sociological Variables

Age

As mentioned previously, older people chose capability cues with greater frequency than any other age group. They also put less reliance on the physician's decision about readiness to go home. Older people have the realistic fear that the inability to care for self could lead to the loss of house or apartment. These factors have implications for the way in which nurses work with older patients.

The meaning and value of self-care differ for each person. It is important, therefore, for nurses to assess self-care needs accurately and assist patients to identify their own values in this area. If the assessment and identification of values for self-care by the nurse differ from that of the patient, there is likely to be conflict. For example, walking with a walker may mean walking for the nurse (after all, the patient is ambulatory), but walking for the patient may mean walking without any aid.

Sometimes nurses use the words "push" or "make" in relation to patient independence. The nurse may make the assessment that the patient is physically capable of doing more for himself or herself. There is the temptation for the nurse to withhold assistance because he or she knows the patient can do more. Withholding help and "making" the patient do something can result in either a compliant or very resistive, angry patient. Once again, goals identified by an individual are more likely to be achieved. With this principle in mind, the nurse could help and support the patient when requested and needed. This support and help can give the patient the sense of security that help is available, and the patient will then feel freer to test out his or her capabilities. Assisting a person to identify his or her own

meaning of self-reliance and offering help when requested
are valid interventions for all patients, especially older ones.
Older patients may have less reserve after major surgery.
They may experience lower energy levels and more depression than younger persons. It is of extreme importance,
therefore, that nurses plan and pace care for the older person with these factors in mind.

Sex

The men in the study did not rate feeling tone cues as
very important. As was pointed out before, this may be a
part of the socialization process for males. Knowing that, at
least for this study, the total group did experience feelings
of depression postsurgery, it would be important for nurses
to convey acceptance of feelings that are expressed by male
patients. Encouraging the expression of feelings requires
skill. Listening and attentiveness to cues the patient is com-
municating can provide the opportunity for the nurse to
help the male patient identify his feelings.

Women, on the other hand, relied on their own feelings and were sensitive to cues from other persons. Again,
this may be a matter of female socialization. As with any
other patient group, it would be important for the nurse to
work with family members and significant others as well as
the patient.

Ethnic group

The Hispanic group showed the greatest difference in
their cues for determining recovery. Cues from family and
friends were very important for this group. Perhaps instead
of viewing family and friends as barriers, nurses could consider family and friends as important in patients' care. Visit-

ing hours could be evaluated by nurses and adjusted according to patients' needs rather than the needs of nurses and other staff. Perhaps also, the nurse can help the patient look to himself or herself, as well as to others.

Although the study data indicated that family and friends were particularly important indicators of recovery for Hispanic patients, it does not follow that family and friends are unimportant for other groups. The support systems available to patients are of great importance in discharge planning. Who is available for shopping, cooking, cleaning, and transportation? The answer to this question is vital, not only for discharge but for the patient's sense of security and his or her recovery process.

Sociological variables were used to see if there were differences among certain groupings of people. The study did demonstrate that these variables had an influence on patient responses. As complex as human beings are, so are the responses of the various people in the study. Therefore, it would be misleading to infer that all persons belonging to a particular group behave in a certain way. The groupings were intended to give insight into how some people within that group behave.

Summary

This study was undertaken to determine the relationship between certain sociological variables and patient's definitions of recovery. Although the study was confined to those persons recovering from abdominal surgery, the results provide interesting insights into the process of recovery from the patient's point of view. The results indicate that the people in the study viewed recovery from a subjective point of view—their capabilities, feelings, and level of strength of energy. For the most part, these are factors that the physician may not consider, and which nurses should consider more fully.

Because of their skills and opportunities for direct patient contact nurses are in a position to work directly with patients in relation to these components of recovery. Further study is indicated to evaluate just how effective nurses are in working with patients on their criteria for recovery. Further study is also needed to include psychological variables and other categories of illness.

Chapter 7

Conclusions and Recommendations

These two studies emphasize that recovery is a process that requires time, energy, and thoughtful attention. The process is not limited to physiological changes, but encompasses psychological changes as well. The recovery process is often given less attention than the acute illness phase, although both are important.

The practice of separating acutely ill and recovering patients has become increasingly widespread, with emphasis on providing the highly skilled and intensive care required during the acute phase. When the patient is transferred from the acute care setting, however, he or she needs different priorities for care, not diminished care or care by less skilled personnel. In many hospitals, units for care of less acutely ill patients largely emphasize the patient's lessened needs for physical care and complicated equipment, without also acknowledging his or her needs for education, counseling, and planning with family, which are especially important for recovering patients.

It is interesting to speculate on the reasons for this difference in emphasis. The needs of acutely ill patients are clear and compelling, while those of recovering patients can

go unnoticed more easily. Idealization of the recovery period, especially among those who can afford it and whose
illness is physical, can interfere with nurses' perceptions of
patients' needs. A patient who is attractively dressed in robe
and slippers, surrounded by flowers and cards, may give
the impression of requiring little of the nurses. One can be
anxious and lonely among the flowers; one can be ill-
informed about self-care though surrounded by greeting
cards. The disparity between the environment of psychiatric
and medical–surgical patients is also striking in this regard.
Psychiatric patients are surrounded less often by these evi-
dences of support from family and friends.

Although nurses concentrate energy on dealing with
crises, it is important to consider some aspects of experience
that are deemphasized during crisis. Leonard Shlain in *Stress
and Survival* (1979) indicates that many people can call upon
coping abilities and support systems during an acute crisis,
and that it is often afterward that the psychological effects of
the experience are most keenly felt. For these people there is
a focusing of energy to deal with the threat during a crisis. In
some instances, of course, the individual is unable to mar-
shall coping abilities, and dissipates energy through severe
anxiety and behavior that interferes with coping, such as
abuse of alcohol. Crisis consumes energy. Frequently other
needs are held in abeyance while energy is directed toward
efforts to resolve the crisis. Feelings such as anger, sadness,
and exhaustion are often experienced after the crisis is over,
feelings the individual may be unaware of during the acute
phase. After the crisis there is opportunity for assessment of
the situation, of what has happened, and of where one
stands. Our culture values the person who moves out of a
crisis "without missing a beat." Such cultural expectations are
unrealistic as many authors, such as Kliman (1978), have
pointed out. People need time to grieve and to come to terms
with changed reality. If this stage is not respected, the indi-

vidual may be burdened with resentment, rage, and fears of caring for himself, which impede his return to functioning as competently as possible, and which may also preclude the personal growth that might otherwise have occurred as as result of the crisis experience.

Nurses' deemphasis on the recovery phase may be related to nurses' view of their role. The nurse's role in supporting and administering treatment to the acutely ill patient has been long acknowledged, and nurses who work with acutely ill clients usually enjoy high professional status. There is less clarity about the role of the nurse in working with the recovering patient. Once physical needs are met (often by an aide) it may seem that there is little else to do. Nursing reports and assignments are illustrative. While the needs of an acutely ill patient may be discussed in detail, care for the patient who is ready to go home is often described in terms such as "There isn't much to do for him. Just make sure his bed is made and that he is taking fluids. He'll be going home tomorrow."

What is the nurse's role in decision making regarding discharge? The Kolditz–Naughton study reported in Chapter 6 points out that the physician is the primary decision maker concerning discharge, and that his or her assessment is based largely on such objective data as laboratory tests. It would be desirable for nurses, patients, and families to have more input into the decision making process. During the course of such collaboration it is important for nurses to be clear about their own values and priorities in relation to patients' discharge, rather than to mirror the physician's views. For instance, the nurse may bring up the issue of a diabetic patient's ability for self-care, while the physician concentrates on blood sugar levels and results of urine tests. Ideally, both professionals would collaborate in their concern for the human aspects of the patient's recovery, but frequently neither physician nor nurse holds this as a high priority.

What can be the role of the nurse who works with

recovering patients? He or she can emphasize planned assessment and intervention that considers the client's needs for counseling and education, as well as for physical care. The way the nurse carries out this role is influenced by his or her view of the recovery process, and by the views of others with whom he or she works. Is recovery viewed primarily as a period of diminishing needs for physical care, or as a dynamic period that presents particular challenges different from but no less important than the acute phase?

Is it part of the nurse's role (as well as the role of other health professionals) to help the client grow emotionally and to learn from experience with illness? If so, she can, for example, help the client who shows readiness to acknowledge the reality of death. She can assist women patients to recognize their own views and become aware of internal cues, as well as turning to others for help. The nurse can provide support and opportunities for expression of feelings when men show "unmanly" behavior such as crying.

Is such a role purely a frill to be offered only when the nurse has extra time? The study by Kolditz and Naughton stresses some important social and economic advantages to skilled assessment and care during recovery. Discharge of a patient before he or she is physically and emotionally ready, or failure to plan adequately for the period following discharge, can lead to readmission, thus increasing costs. Patients who fail to achieve maximum recovery, although not readmitted, represent a social and personal loss that can extend for years, limiting their functioning as individuals, family members, and workers. As an example, there are stroke patients who receive adequate care during the acute phase, only to be discharged with inadequate plans for care during the lengthy recovery phase, and who remain unnecessarily disabled.

It is widely acknowledged that much of the recovery process occurs after discharge from an acute care setting. However, the adequacy of the patient's support system often remains unexplored when he or she leaves the hospital. The recent focus in nursing has been on initial assessment upon entry to the hospital. Equally careful assessment of family, home environment, and other aspects of the patient's situation is necessary prior to discharge. It is essential to remember that the patient's family and work environments are ongoing systems that change during the course of his or her absence. The patient may find that he or she is in a situation similar to trying to jump aboard a moving carousel, rather than being assisted aboard, unless thoughtful care is given to his or her reentry into family and work life. For many patients, care following discharge is limited largely to periodic visits to the physician or clinic, where attention often is focused on objective data and little attention is given to their human responses to the illness and their reentry into work and family life. While some nurses are providing care to these patients through private practice and community health nursing, many patients lack necessary nursing care during this period. A key concern involves the independence of nurses. If nurses are viewed largely as assistants to the physician, it follows that they will limit their care to carrying out various tasks that the physician delegates. If, however, nurses are viewed as having an independent sphere of practice, it is appropriate that they concern themselves with those aspects of care which they themselves note and with which they are prepared to deal. Readiness for discharge is one such aspect. It would be appropriate for nurses to assume a major role in this area and to refer patients to other nurses, such as to those in private practice or in community health nursing for follow-up care when they themselves cannot provide it. This view has been expressed for many years; nevertheless, the actual decision making concerning discharge and postdischarge care has remained largely the province of physicians.

Nursing has spoken to the necessity for maintaining

and rekindling abilities for self-help. Institutional policies and some health care personnel, however, sometimes forget these needs. Patients who can carry out as much of their own physical care as possible can thereby increase confidence in themselves and at the same time lessen the debilitating effects of unnecessary immobility. Many surgical patients only briefly lose their ability to take a shower, wear comfortable lounge clothes, and sit at a table for meals. Often the night dress, bed tray, and bath basin routines continue throughout the hospital stay, not because patients need it, but because these measures are applied to all patients regardless of their suitability.

While these considerations are important for all patients, they are especially so for geriatric patients. The study by Kolditz and Naughton indicates that geriatric patients are the least influenced by the views of others regarding cues for recovery and that they are very concerned about such internal cues as their own energy and capability for self-care. It is likely that in a culture in which a faltering older person is quickly consigned indefinitely to a custodial institution, the older individual may feel very threatened by any illness that could precipitate such an event. Measures that help the patient maintain physical abilities and confidence are especially necessary, therefore, for older clients. There is a tendency among health care professionals to ignore older clients' views of their abilities. Staff often turn to the family to make decisions, leaving the patient out of the process. Thus, there is a contradiction between the client's tendency to rely on his or her inner cues and staff's tendency to disregard the client's views and to focus instead on others' views of the client's abilities.

Many of the patients in the study by Smith (Chapters 3–5) were middle class. Therefore, when they were asked about priorities and values, responses were undoubtedly affected by middle-class values. Had patients of other classes been more fully represented, perhaps other values would have been cited. Since caregivers also tend to be middle class, it may be that it is easier for them to recognize and appreciate the values of these patients, and that particularly attentive listening and recognition of one's own biases may be necessary when working with patients with different backgrounds.

What is there in this for nurses besides the recognition that patients benefit from their knowledge and skills? Howard Kogan, a contributor to *Stress and Survival* (1979), points out that caregivers experience personal growth, too, as they assist patients to confront survival issues. Unfortunately, many nurses are confined to routine tasks, which deprive not only their clients but themselves of the rewards that could be theirs through more independent, creative practice.

Many patients are confronting fundamental issues of life and death and of the quality and purpose of life—issues that are frequently obscured by daily preoccupations. The nurse who develops the skills and sensitivity to tune in to patients' existential concerns has an opportunity for personal growth that continues as long as he or she works with patients. This is a humanizing influence on nursing practice, that provides nurses with a depth and richness of experience that may be denied to those nurses who limit themselves to the performance of routine tasks. The nurse frequently comes away from contact with a patient feeling more sure of values and priorities. The patient's care was not just a job to be done; it was an experience of growth, insight, a surer sense of reality, and a deepened appreciation of the gift of life. In such moments the nurse often realizes that he or she gave and received a great deal during that experience with the patient. Thus nurses are touched, as survivors are touched, by the fundamental facts of existence. In this touching there is a freeing of potential for growth. Just as patients are frequently not the same as before as survival experience, nurses, too, are not the same after a "touching" experience involving the care and nurture of another person. Through such experiences, for patients and for those who care for them, life is enriched.

References and Selected Readings

Acquilera, D. et al. *Crisis Intervention.* St. Louis: C.V. Mosby, 1970.

Antonovsky, Aaron. *Health Stress and Coping.* San Francisco: Jossey-Bass, 1979.

Bettelheim, Bruno. *The Informed Heart.* Glencoe, Ill.: Free Press, 1960.

Bilodeau, C. B., and Hackett, T. P. "Issues raised in a group setting by patients recovering from myocardial infarction," *American Journal of Psychiatry* 128: 73–78, 1971.

Booth, Gotthard. "Psychobiological aspects of spontaneous regressions of cancer," *Journal of the American Academy of Psychoanalysis* 1:303–307, 1973.

Burgess, Ann, and Lazare, Aaron. *Psychiatric Nursing in the Hospital and Community.* Englewood Cliffs, N.J.: Prentice-Hall, 1973.

Camus, Albert. *The Plague* (transl. by S. Gilbert). New York: Random House, 1948.

Carlson, Carolyn. "Grief and Mourning." In *Behavioral Concepts and Nursing Interventions,* coordinated by Carolyn Carlson. Philadelphia: J.B. Lippincott, 1970.

Des Pres, Terrence. *The Survivor.* New York: Oxford University Press, 1976.

Dimsdale, Joel. "Coping: Every Man's War," *American Journal of Psychotherapy* 32:402, 1978.

Erikson, Kai T. *Everything in Its Path.* New York: Simon and Schuster, 1976.

Frankl, Viktor E. *From Death Camp to Existentialism*. Boston: Beacon Press, 1959.

Garfield, Charles, ed. *Stress and Survival*. St. Louis: C.V. Mosby, 1979.

Handlin, Oscar. *The Uprooted*, 2d ed. Boston: Little, Brown, 1973.

Hitchcock, T. A. "Crisis Intervention," *American Journal of Nursing* 73:1388, August 1973.

Hollingshead, August B. *Two-factor Index of Social Position*. 1957 (mimeograph).

Horowitz, Mardi. *Stress Response Syndromes*. New York: Jason Aronson, 1976.

Howard, Stephen. "The Vietnam Warrior," *American Journal of Psychotherapy* 30:121, January 1976.

Jung, C. G. *Psychological Reflections*. Ed. by Jolande Jacobi. New York: Harper & Row, 1953.

Jungk, Robert. *Children of the Ashes*. New York: Harcourt, Brace, 1961.

Kliman, Ann S. *Crisis: Psychological First Aid for Recovery and Growth*. New York: Holt, Rinehart, & Winston, 1978.

Kogan, Howard. "A Therapist Encounters the Possibility of an Early Death." In *Stress and Survival*. Ed. by Charles Garfield. St. Louis: C.V. Mosby, 1979.

Kohn, Melvin. *Social Class and Conformity*. Homewood, Ill.: Dorsey Press, 1969.

Koos, Earl L. *The Health of Regionville*. New York: Columbia University Press, 1954.

Kübler-Ross, Elisabeth. *On Death and Dying*. New York: Macmillan, 1969.

LeShan, Lawrence. "Cancer and Personality," *Journal of the National Cancer Institute* 22:1–18, 1959.

Lifton, Robert J. *Home from the War*. New York: Simon & Schuster, 1973.

———. *Living and Dying*. New York: Praeger, 1974.

———. *History and Human Survival*. New York: Vantage Books, 1976.

Lindemann, Erich. "Symptomatology and Management of Grief." In *Crisis Intervention*, ed. by Howard J. Parad. New York: Family Service Association of America, 1965.

Maloney, Elizabeth M. "Subjective and Objective Definition of Crisis," *Perspectives in Psychiatric Care* 9:259, November–December 1971.

Marram, Gwen D. *The Group Approach in Nursing Practice*. St. Louis: C.V. Mosby, 1973.

Maslow, A. H. *The Farther Reaches of Human Nature*. New York: Viking, 1971.

Mechanic, David. *Medical Sociology: A Selective View*. Glencoe, Ill.: Free Press, 1968.

Mitscherlich, Alexander, and Mitscherlich, Margarete. *The Inability to Mourn* (transl. by Beverly R. Placzek). New York: Grove Press, 1975.

Muhlen, Norbert. *The Survivors*. New York: T.Y. Crowell, 1962.

Neiderland, W. "The Problem of the Survivor," *Journal of the Hillside Hospital* 10:233, 1961.

Parad, Howard. *Crisis Intervention*. New York: Family Service Association of America, 1965.

Parkes, C. M. *Bereavement: Studies of Grief in Adult Life*. New York: International Universities Press, 1972.

Parsons, Talcott. "Definitions of Health and Illness in the Light of American Values and Social Structure." In *Patients, Physician and Illness*. Ed. by E. Gartley Jaco. New York: The Free Press, 1972.

Phillips, Russell E. "Impact of Nazi Holocaust on children of survivors," *American Journal of Psychotherapy* 32:370, July 1978.

Rubenstein, Richard L. *After Auschwitz*. New York: Bobbs Merrill, 1966.

Saunders, Lyle. *Cultural Differences and Medical Care*. New York: Russell Sage, 1954.

Shlain, Leonard. "Cancer Is Not a Four Letter Word." In *Stress and Survival*. Ed. by Charles Garfield. St. Louis: C.V. Mosby, 1979.

Simonton, O.C. "Management of Emotional Aspects of Malignancy." In *New Dimensions of Habilitation for the Handicapped*. Gainesville: University of Florida Press, 1974.

Smith, Dorothy W. "Patienthood and Its Threat to Privacy," *American Journal of Nursing* 69:508–513, March 1969.

Stillman, Margot J. "Territoriality and Personal Space," *American Journal of Nursing* 78:1670–1672, October 1978.

Zborowski, Mark. *People in Pain*. San Francisco: Jossey-Bass, 1969.

Index